Myocardial Infarction

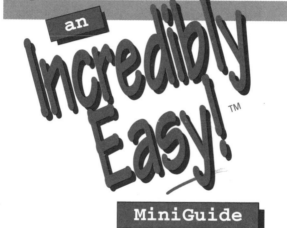

an **Incredibly Easy!**™

MiniGuide

Myocardial Infarction

an

Incredibly Easy!™

MiniGuide

Springhouse Corporation
Springhouse, Pennsylvania

Staff

Vice President
Matthew Cahill

Clinical Director
Judith A. Schilling McCann,
RN, MSN

Art Director
John Hubbard

Executive Editor
Michael Shaw

Managing Editor
Andrew T. McPhee, RN,
BSN

Clinical Editors
Joan M. Robinson, RN,
MSN, CCRN (clinical project
manager); Jill Curry, RN,
BSN; Carla M. Roy, RN,
BSN, CCRN; Gwynn
Sinkinson, RN,C, NP

Editors
Kevin Haworth, Edward R.
Pratowski

Copy Editors
Brenna H. Mayer (manager),
Priscilla DeWitt, Stacey Ann
Follin, Pamela Wingrod

Designers
Arlene Putterman (associ-
ate art director), Mary
Ludwicki (book designer),
Joseph John Clark, Donna
S. Morris, Jacalyn B.
Facciolo

Illustrator
Bot Roda, Betty Winnberg

Typography
Diane Paluba (manager),
Joyce Rossi Biletz, Valerie
Molettiere

Manufacturing
Deborah Meiris (director),
Patricia K. Dorshaw (man-
ager), Otto Mezei (book pro-
duction manager)

Editorial Assistants
Beverly Lane, Marcia Mills,
Liz Schaeffer

Indexer
Ellen Murray

The clinical treatments described
and recommended in this publica-
tion are based on research and
consultation with nursing, medical,
and legal authorities. To the best of
our knowledge, these procedures
reflect currently accepted practice.
Nevertheless, they can't be considered absolute and universal recommendations. For individual applica-
tions, all recommendations must be
considered in light of the patient's
clinical condition and, before
administration of new or infre-
quently used drugs, in light of the
latest package-insert information.
The authors and the publisher dis-
claim any responsibility for any
adverse effects resulting from the
suggested procedures, from any
undetected errors, or from the
reader's misunderstanding of the
text.

Printed in the United States of
America

IEMMI-010899

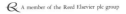 A member of the Reed Elsevier plc group

```
Library of Congress Cataloging-in-
Publication Data

Myocardial infarction: an incredibly
  easy miniguide
      p.  cm.—(Miniguides)
      Includes index.
      1. Myocardial infarction
Handbooks, manuals, etc. I.
Springhouse Corporation. II.
Series: Incredibly easy miniguide.
[DNLM: 1. Myocardial Infarction
Handbooks. WG 39 M997 1999]
RC685.1'237—dc21
DNLM/DLC                       99-32918
ISBN 1-58255-009-3 (alk. paper)  CIP
```

Contents

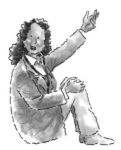

Contributors and consultants

Joanne M. Bartelmo, RN, MSN, CCRN
Clinical Educator
Pottstown (Pa.) Memorial
Medical Center

Nancy Cirone, RN,C, MSN, CDE
Director of Education
Warminster (Pa.) Hospital

Margaret Friant Cramer, RN, MSN
Clinical Supervisor
Cardiac Solutions, Inc.
Fort Washington, Pa.

Michael Carter, RN, DNSc, FAAN
Dean and Professor
College of Nursing
University of Tennessee
Memphis

Pamela Mullen Kovach, RN, BSN
Independent Clinical
Consultant
Perkiomenville, Pa.

Patricia A. Lange, RN, MSN, EdD (candidate), **CS, CCRN**
Graduate Nursing Program
Coordinator and Assistant
Professor of Nursing
Hawaii Pacific University
Kaneohe

Mary Ann Siciliano McLaughlin, RN, MSN
Clinical Supervisor
Cardiac Solutions, Inc.
Fort Washington, Pa.

Lori Musolf Neri, RN, MSN, CCRN
Clinical Instructor
Villanova (Pa.) University

Joseph L. Neri, DO, FACC
Cardiologist
The Heart Care Group
Allentown, Pa.

Robert Rauch
Manager of Government
Economics
Amgen, Inc.
Thousand Oaks, Calif.

Larry E. Simmons, RN, PhD (candidate)
Clinical Instructor
University of Missouri-
Kansas City

Foreword

Few conditions inspire fear in a patient like myocardial infarction. As a health care professional on the front lines of the battle against MI, you must have the information at your fingertips to treat the disorder effectively and to address your patient's concerns about prevention and recovery. It's a tough job, but now you're holding in your hands something that can help.

The clinical experts at Springhouse have created *Myocardial Infarction: An Incredibly Easy MiniGuide,* a revolutionary new MI patient care reference. This handy book will help you gain an understanding of MI in an unusually off-beat, up-lifting, easy-going way, without ever sacrificing accuracy or thoroughness.

The first chapter, *Understanding MI,* establishes a basis for excellent patient care by reviewing the steps that lead to MI. The second chapter follows with an in-depth discussion of MI risk factors. The next three chapters cover assessment, treatment, and complications. The final chapter covers patient teaching and provides an up-to-date list of further references available by telephone and on the internet.

Throughout the book, you'll find special features designed to strengthen your understanding of MI and its effects on your patient. *Checklists,* rendered in the style of a classroom chalkboard, provide at-a-glance summaries of important facts, while *Memory joggers* provide clever tricks for remembering key points.

The book also features cartoon characters throughout that provide light-hearted chuckles while they reinforce essential material. And a *Quick quiz* at the end of every chapter helps you assess your learning and refresh your memory at the same time.

You'll be amazed at the amount of information contained in this truly pocket-size guide. If you want an easy-to-read, comprehensive reference about one of today's most serious health care issues, I can't think of a better resource than *Myocardial Infarction: An Incredibly Easy MiniGuide*. It's truly a pint-size powerhouse.

Michael Carter, RN, DNSc, FAAN
Dean and Professor
College of Nursing
University of Tennessee
Memphis

> Finally, an MI reference that will never be far from your fingertips.

1

Understanding MI

> ### Key facts
> ◆ In a myocardial infarction (MI), a portion of the heart's myocardium is damaged.
> ◆ Most commonly, an MI occurs when normal blood flow to the heart is decreased.
> ◆ Reduced blood flow usually results from a thrombus in the coronary artery.

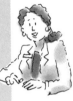

Pathophysiology

In most cases, an MI occurs when normal blood flow to the heart decreases. Decreased blood flow usually results from blockage with a thrombus in a coronary artery. It may also result from:
• coronary artery spasm
• embolism in a coronary artery
• sudden drop in blood pressure during surgery.

Too much demand

In other cases, the heart's need for oxygen increases beyond what the blood flow can supply. Causes of increased demand include:

- cocaine abuse
- heavy exertion
- increase in catecholamine levels
- stress
- sudden increase in blood pressure.

Another brick in the wall

An MI affects the wall of the heart. The wall of the heart is made up of three layers of cardiac tissue. The myocardium is the middle, striated muscle layer and the thickest layer of the heart wall. The myocardium is the layer affected during an MI.

The art of the arteries

The heart receives blood from a system of coronary arteries. This system includes the right and left main coronary arteries. The left main coronary artery divides into the left anterior descending and the left circumflex arteries. The right coronary artery turns down the back of the heart, becoming the posterior descending artery. (See *Viewing coronary vessels.*)

> Oh my, my myocardium, my middle muscular layer. It's the layer affected during an MI.

Viewing coronary vessels

The illustration below shows the major coronary vessels.

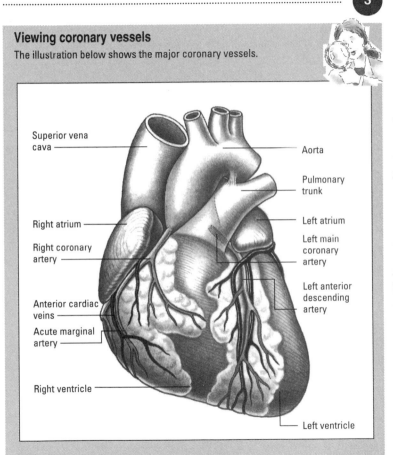

- Superior vena cava
- Aorta
- Pulmonary trunk
- Right atrium
- Left atrium
- Right coronary artery
- Left main coronary artery
- Left anterior descending artery
- Anterior cardiac veins
- Acute marginal artery
- Right ventricle
- Left ventricle

Now I get it!

Factors affecting myocardial damage

If an occlusion in a coronary artery causes an MI, the amount of damage to the myocardium depends on three factors:

👆 the area of the heart supplied by the affected vessel

✌️ the demand for oxygen in the affected area of the heart

🖖 the collateral circulation in the affected area of the heart. (Collateral circulation is an alternative circulation, which develops when blood flow to a tissue is blocked.)

Location, location, location

An MI's severity depends partly on the location of the blockage in the coronary artery. Because blood is denied to a larger area of the myocardium, a blockage located higher in the artery can cause more damage. (See *Factors affecting myocardial damage*.)

Occlusion may occur in an artery that supplies blood to the heart. The specific artery that becomes occluded also af-

Sites of occlusion

The chart below links areas of the heart wall that may be affected during MI with sites of coronary artery occlusion.

Wall affected during an MI	Sight of occlusion
Inferior wall	Right coronary artery
Lateral wall	Circumflex artery, branch of the left anterior descending artery
Anterior wall	Left coronary artery, left anterior descending artery
Posterior wall	Right coronary artery, circumflex artery
Anterolateral wall	Left anterior descending artery, circumflex artery
Anteroseptal wall	Left anterior descending artery

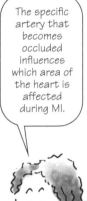

The specific artery that becomes occluded influences which area of the heart is affected during MI.

fects which area of the heart is affected during an MI. (See *Sites of occlusion*.)

Right ventricular infarction

Most commonly an MI occurs in the left ventricle. However, a patient can develop an MI in the right ventricle or in both ventricles.

A right ventricular infarction develops from blockage in the right coronary artery (which supplies the right ventricle and the lower left ventricle) and involves the inferior wall.

Ischemia, injury, infarction

When blood supply fails to meet the myocardium's demand, the myocardium suffers progressive damage. Damage begins in the subendocardium and extends toward the epicardium. The types of tissue damage (referred to as zones of tissue damage) in an early acute MI are ischemia, injury, and infarction. (See *Zones of tissue damage in MI.*)

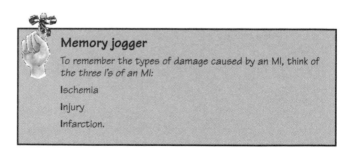

Memory jogger

To remember the types of damage caused by an MI, think of the three I's of an MI:

Ischemia

Injury

Infarction.

Now I get it!

Zones of tissue damage in MI

When the myocardium is deprived of an oxygen-rich blood supply, three types of pathological changes may occur: ischemia, injury, and infarction (also known as myocardial necrosis).

Zone of ischemia
The outermost area is the zone of ischemia. Ischemia results from an interrupted blood supply.

Zone of injury
Injury results from a prolonged lack of blood supply. The zone of injury surrounds the zone of infarction.

Zone of infarction
Infarction is also known as myocardial necrosis. Eventually, the dead tissue is replaced by scar tissue. Injury and ischemia are reversible, if treatment begins promptly. Necrosis isn't reversible.

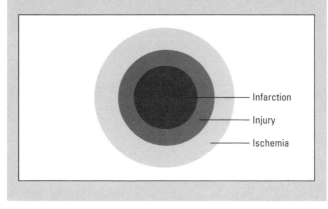

Effects of MI

Myocardial damage limits the heart's ability to function properly. Depending on which coronary artery is affected, damage may extend to the conduction system, leading to decreased cardiac output and arrhythmias.

Pain plus

The pain associated with an MI is caused by the death of myocardial tissue. The pain, usually in the chest, can also be referred to the neck, jaw, back, or left arm. This pain will last more than a few minutes or will go away and come back.

> The pain associated with MI is caused by the death of myocardial tissue.

Other common signs and symptoms

The patient may also exhibit:
- dyspnea
- fainting
- hypotension
- light-headedness
- nausea or vomiting
- sweating.

What happens in MI *(continued)*

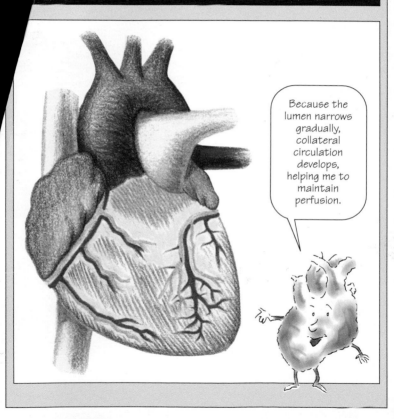

What happens in MI

It all begins in the coronary arteries, where an injury to an artery's lining causes platelets, white blood cells, fibrin, and lipids to converge at the injured site.

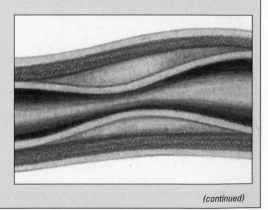

Foam cells, or resident macrophages, then congregate under the damaged lining and absorb oxidized cholesterol, forming a fatty streak that narrows the arterial lumen and reduces the heart's blood supply.

(continued)

What happens in MI (continued)

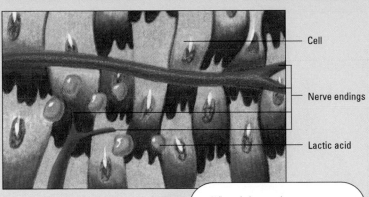

Cell

Nerve endings

Lactic acid

When I demand more oxygen than collateral circulation can supply, myocardial metabolism shifts from aerobic to anaerobic, producing lactic acid.

(continued)

What happens in MI *(continued)*

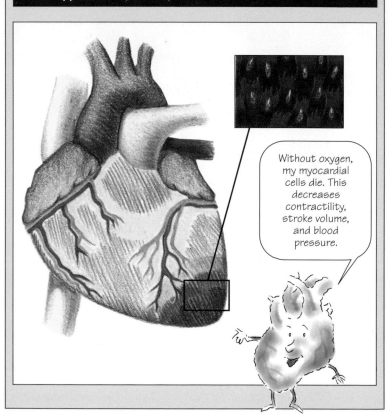

Without oxygen, my myocardial cells die. This decreases contractility, stroke volume, and blood pressure.

What happens in MI *(continued)*

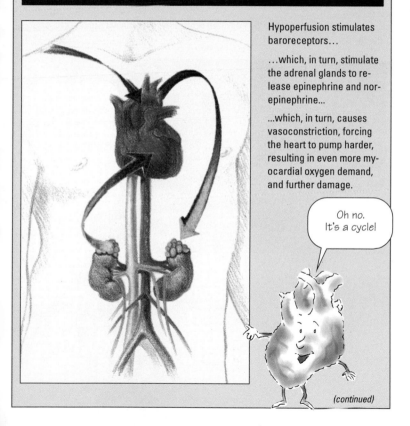

Hypoperfusion stimulates baroreceptors...

...which, in turn, stimulate the adrenal glands to release epinephrine and norepinephrine...

...which, in turn, causes vasoconstriction, forcing the heart to pump harder, resulting in even more myocardial oxygen demand, and further damage.

Oh no. It's a cycle!

(continued)

What happens in MI *(continued)*

Damaged cell membranes in the infarcted area allow intracellular contents to leak into the vascular circulation.

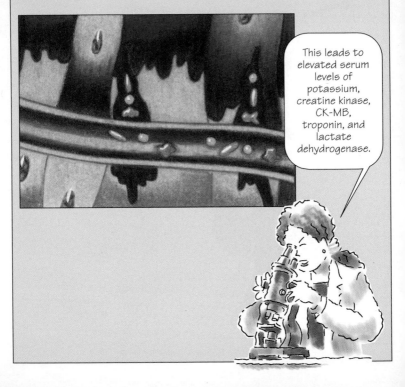

This leads to elevated serum levels of potassium, creatine kinase, CK-MB, troponin, and lactate dehydrogenase.

What happens in MI (continued)

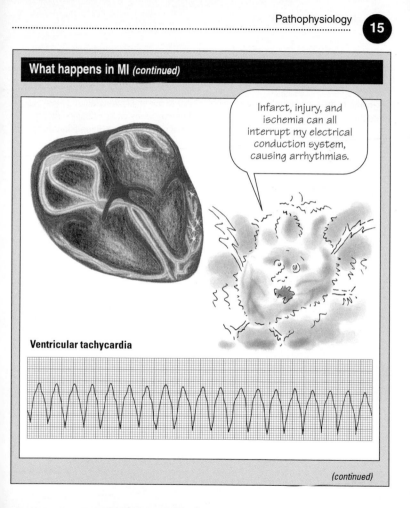

Ventricular tachycardia

(continued)

What happens in MI *(continued)*

Damage to the left ventricle may impair its ability to pump, allowing blood to back up into the left atrium and, eventually, into the pulmonary veins and capillaries. As the back pressure rises, fluid crosses the alveolocapillary membrane, impeding the diffusion of oxygen and carbon dioxide. As a consequence, the patient may develop heart failure.

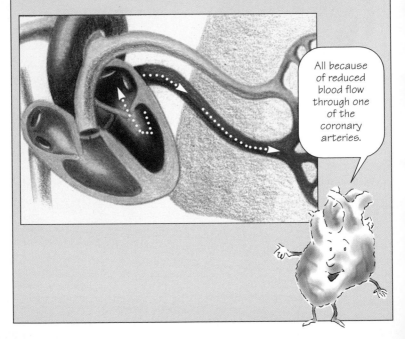

ECG changes

If the myocardium is deprived of an oxy-gen-rich blood supply, pathologic changes will be reflected on an electro-cardiogram (ECG). Certain ECG find-ings are characteristic of an MI:
• ST-segment elevation
• large, inverted T waves
• large, pathologic Q waves. (For more about ECG changes, see chapter 3, Assessing patients with MI.)

Q wave or non–Q wave MI

The presence or absence of pathologic Q waves may be used to describe the specific type of MI. In Q-wave (transmur-al) MI, tissue damage extends through all myocardial layers. In non–Q-wave (subendocardial) MI, usually only the in-nermost layer is damaged.

Prognosis

Rapid treatment can prevent myocardial necrosis. If symptoms persist for more than 6 hours, little can be done to pre-vent necrosis. Therefore, administering medical care as soon as the patient's symptoms begin is crucial.

Quick quiz

1. The most common cause of an MI is:

    A. coronary artery spasm.

    B. coronary emboli.

    C. coronary artery thrombus.

Answer: C. Coronary artery thrombus is the most common cause of an MI.

2. The three zones of tissue damage in an early acute MI are all reversible except:

    A. ischemia.

    B. injury.

    C. infarction.

Answer: C. Infarction (also called necrosis) isn't reversible. Injury and ischemia are reversible, if treatment begins promptly.

Scoring

☆☆☆ If you answered both questions correctly, my-oh-my! You're managing myocardial matters magnificently.

☆☆ If you answered fewer than two questions correctly, keep studying. You'll be pumping out quick quiz answers in a heartbeat.

Preventing MI

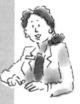

Key facts
◆ Patients exhibit both modifiable and non-modifiable risk factors that may predispose them to a myocardial infarction (MI).

◆ Identifying nonmodifiable risk factors may help to motivate your patient to seek early treatment or take other preventive steps.

◆ Factors that can be modified to reduce the risk of an MI include a sedentary lifestyle, smoking, hyperlipidemia, hypertension, diabetes, cocaine use, and obesity.

◆ If a patient has coronary artery disease, steps to prevent an MI may include nitroglycerin, aspirin, or a beta-adrenergic blocker.

MI risk

The first step in prevention is to evaluate a person's risk for an MI. Risk factors for an MI may or may not be modifiable.

Nonmodifiable risk factors

Although certain risk factors can't be changed, identifying them may help mo-

tivate your patient to seek early treatment or take other preventive steps. Risk factors that can't be modified include:
- age (men over 55, women over 65)
- family history of an MI
- gender (men more at risk)
- genetic predisposition to high cholesterol level
- race (blacks more at risk)
- history of angina pectoris.

Age

Risk for an MI increases steadily as a patient ages. Four out of five people who die of an MI are age 65 or older.

All in the family

Increased risk for MI depends on which members of a patient's family suffered an MI and when. A patient's risk of MI increases if:
- his mother had an MI before menopause
- his father had an MI before age 50 or didn't survive his first MI
- his sibling had an MI before age 55.

Men after age 45, women after menopause

Though MI may occur at any age, men usually experience an MI after age 45.

Women usually have their first MI after menopause. Until then, estrogen helps protect women's hearts from MI.

Familial hypercholesterolemia

Some patients have a genetic predisposition to high cholesterol, which increases the risk of MI. Familial hypercholesterolemia is an inherited metabolic disorder, caused by defective or absent low-density lipoprotein (LDL) receptors on cell surfaces. This results in an increase in blood plasma LDL and an accumulation of LDL in the body. Familial hypercholesterolemia is a dominant genetic trait, so a person only needs to inherit one abnormal gene to develop this condition.

A person only needs to inherit one abnormal gene to develop familial hypercholesterolemia.

Race and hypertension

Ethnicity influences a person's risk for an MI because of the link between hypertension and MI.

Hypertension is two to three times more common in blacks than in whites; therefore, blacks are three times more likely to experience a cardiac death and two times more likely to experience a nonfatal MI.

Because the risk of an MI is increased, blacks with hypertension are urged to stay physically active and follow a low-fat diet. Because hypertension is a familial disorder, family members should also exercise, eat right, and get regular checkups.

Modifiable risk factors

By taking steps to change factors that put them at risk, patients can reduce their risk of coronary artery disease (CAD) and significantly lower their chances of experiencing an MI. Modifiable factors include:
- cocaine use
- diabetes
- hyperlipidemia
- hypertension
- obesity
- sedentary lifestyle
- smoking.

Advice from the experts

Stress, alcohol, and MI

Stress or alcohol use may cause the heart (and other organs) to work harder. Over time, stress or alcohol use may eventually wear down the heart, increasing the risk of heart disease and hypertension.

I'll drink to that

Alcohol slows down the central nervous system (CNS), but this effect isn't as restful as it seems. Frequent or excessive alcohol use progressively increases blood pressure and thus adds to the workload of the heart. The patient should limit daily intake to one of the following:
• less than 24 oz (710 ml) of beer
• 8 oz (235 ml) of wine
• 2 oz (60 ml) of hard liquor.

Run rabbit run

Stress speeds up the CNS, activating the sympathetic nervous system. Chronic stress doesn't allow the body enough time to recover. Damage to organs, including the heart, results from exhaustion.

Mellow out

The way a person tends to react to stressful situations may be related to coronary artery disease (CAD). People whose heart rates and blood pressure increase a great deal when they're exposed to a frustrating situation may be more likely to develop CAD.

Stress and excessive alcohol intake are considered possible risk factors. (See *Stress, alcohol, and MI.*)

Cancel the coke

Cocaine use adds to the risk of heart disease. It elevates blood pressure, causes arrhythmia, leads to vasoconstriction, and may speed up atherosclerosis. If cocaine is used in combination with alcohol and cigarette smoking, the incidence of cardiac death increases dramatically.

The effect cocaine has on the body varies with each individual, because the drug itself varies in strength, dose, and method of ingestion. First-time users as well as regular users are at risk for all of the harmful effects.

> Silence can be deadly. A silent MI occurs without chest pain.

Deal with diabetes

Because of the neurologic deficits that accompany uncontrolled hyperglycemia, diabetic patients are at risk for a silent MI. A silent MI occurs without the chest pain that is typically associated with an MI. The patient may feel like he has a cold or flu or may not experience any discomfort.

A patient is usually unaware of a silent MI, until a routine electrocardiogram detects an old MI or the patient develops heart failure.

To help control diabetes, encourage the patient to do the following:
• Take insulin or an oral antidiabetic drug, as ordered.
• Monitor the blood glucose level regularly.
• Continue regular checkups and follow-up care.

Cut cholesterol

Cholesterol is a fatty protein manufactured by the liver. A high cholesterol level, or hyperlipidemia, is defined as a total cholesterol level over 200 mg/dl. (For more information on cholesterol levels, see *Understanding cholesterol,* page 26.)

A genetic tendency toward high cholesterol can't be altered; however, patients can reduce the total cholesterol level by watching their diets, using antilipemics (if prescribed), and exercising regularly. Taking these steps can help lower the risk of early cardiac problems.

Halt hypertension

Hypertension is defined as a systolic blood pressure over 140 mm Hg or a diastolic blood pressure over 90 mm Hg for

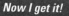

Now I get it!

Understanding cholesterol

A blood cholesterol reading reflects the amount of cholesterol circulating in the bloodstream.

The good and the bad

Different kinds of cholesterol exist. High-density lipoprotein (HDL) cholesterol is considered "good" cholesterol because it removes excess cholesterol from the circulatory system. Low-density lipoprotein (LDL) cholesterol is considered "bad" cholesterol because it collects in artery walls and contributes to the development of atherosclerotic plaque. Cholesterol tests commonly measure triglycerides (blood fats) along with HDL and LDL.

Recommended cholesterol levels

Primary goals:
- If the patient has less than two risk factors for MI, that patient's LDL level should be less than 160 mg/dl.
- If the patient has two or more risk factors, LDL level should be less than 130 mg/dl.

Secondary goals:
- The patient's HDL level should be greater than 35 mg/dl.
- The patient's triglyceride level should be less than 200 mg/dl.

three consecutive readings. The higher the blood pressure, the harder the heart has to work to eject blood from the left ventricle.

Over time, uncontrolled hypertension significantly increases the heart's workload. This increased workload can also cause left ventricle hypertrophy.

To control hypertension, instruct the patient to do the following:

• Continue taking the prescribed antihypertensive, unless otherwise directed.

• Exercise every day.

• Lose weight.

• Continue regular checkups and follow-up care.

• Limit salt intake.

Watching weight

Obesity increases the workload of the heart and the risk of CAD and hypertension. To reduce weight, patients should do the following:

• Maintain a low-fat, low-cholesterol diet. (See *Lowering cholesterol,* p 28.)

• Exercise regularly.

Get off the couch

Patients with sedentary lifestyles place themselves at increased risk for MI. To stay fit, the heart needs a minimum of 20 minutes of continuous cardiovascular

To stay fit, I need a minimum of 20 minutes of continuous cardiovascular exercise three times a week.

Lowering cholesterol

The first step in helping the patient reduce cholesterol is to encourage a low-fat, low-cholesterol diet emphasizing fruits, vegetables, and fish.

Healthy recommendations

Give your patients the following advice:
- Eat a wide variety of foods for a healthy diet.
- Use low-fat dairy products.
- Choose lean meat, such as chicken or turkey.
- Trim the fat from meat, and remove skin from poultry.
- Use unsaturated vegetable oils and margarine instead of butter.
- Limit intake of saturated fat and high-fat products.
- Check all labels for information on fat and carbohydrates.
- Plan meals in advance. Fast food usually isn't healthy enough.
- Shop when you're not hungry. You'll make wiser decisions.
- Broil, bake, grill, or steam food. Don't fry it.
- Eat more fruits, vegetables, and grains.
- Eat a big breakfast, moderate lunch, and small dinner.
- Eat low-fat, low-sugar cereal.
- Eliminate soda and other high-sugar drinks.
- Drink about a half-gallon of water every day.
- Exercise at least a little bit every day.

No replacement for diet

If dietary changes fail to reduce cholesterol, the doctor may prescribe an antilipemic to help the patient maintain a safer cholesterol level. Dietary restrictions must continue during drug therapy. The patient should take antilipemics in the evening to decrease adverse reactions.

exercise (exercise that elevates the heart rate) three times per week. (See *Teaching about exercise,* page 30.)

Say no to nicotine

Smoking exposes the body to nicotine, which has several negative effects on the heart. These effects include vasoconstriction of the coronary arteries and loss of smoothness along the arteries' intima. Encourage the patient to stop smoking. Many resources are available to help the patient. (See *Quitting smoking,* pages 31 and 32.)

If a patient develops CAD, following guidelines for modifiable risk factors becomes even more important.

Preventing MI in patients with CAD

A patient with CAD may take steps to reduce the risk of an MI and prevent sudden cardiac death.

If a patient develops CAD, it becomes even more important to follow guidelines for modifiable risk factors. Because of the increased risk, you should familiarize the patient with the warning signs of an

(Text continues on page 32.)

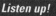

Listen up!

Teaching about exercise

Here are some tips and guidelines you can share with your patient to help him find the right exercise program and stick with it.

Aerobic or anaerobic

Aerobic exercise increases the heart rate and respiratory rate. Such exercise builds cardiovascular endurance but usually does little to build muscle mass. Walking and swimming are aerobic.

Anaerobic exercise involves short bursts of activity, usually against a resistance. Such exercises strengthen muscles but don't necessarily improve cardiovascular endurance. Weight training is anaerobic.

Benefits of exercise

Exercise can help your patient change every modifiable risk factor, greatly reducing the chances of MI.

Increased good cholesterol

Exercise can raise the level of high-density lipoprotein, or good cholesterol, by 5% to 15%.

Pressure drop

After exercise, people with moderate hypertension experience a drop (of 10 to 14 mm Hg) in systolic blood pressure.

Less stress

Exercise reduces stress by removing the person from a stressful environment, increasing energy level, and releasing mood-improving endorphins.

Other benefits

Exercise can help patients with diabetes lower blood glucose levels and increase insulin sensitivity. Exercise also aids in smoking cessation.

Listen up!

Quitting smoking

Regardless of the method your patient uses to quit, the urge to smoke will never completely go away. This can be discouraging. Tell the patient that the urge to smoke does decrease, however, after 7 days of abstinence.

Methods of quitting

Your patients may use one or more of the techniques listed below.

Exercise

Regular exercise will clear the lungs, get the internal organs in shape, and decrease the ex-smoker's weight gain by increasing the metabolism (naturally).

Nicotine patches

Nicotine patches suppress the symptoms of nicotine withdrawal by delivering a continuous trickle of nicotine through the skin. People shouldn't smoke while using the patch.

Nicotine gum

This gum suppresses withdrawal symptoms by administering nicotine in a sugar-free gum. Whenever a craving strikes, the person can chew a piece of gum for approximately ½ hour. People should never exceed 30 pieces of gum per day.

Bupropion

Bupropion (Zyban) is a nicotine-free prescription antidepressant. When used in low doses, this drug has been more effective than nicotine replacement therapy. People can use this drug along with nicotine patches or gum, but it may interact with other drugs.

(continued)

MI. To reduce the heart's workload, the patient may take medications, such as nitroglycerin, aspirin, and beta-adrenergic blockers.

Nitroglycerin

Nitroglycerin helps to decrease the workload of the heart and allows the heart to meet its oxygen needs.

Patients with CAD may take oral nitrates, such as Isordil and Imdur, daily to prevent angina attacks. Patients may take sublingual nitroglycerin, as needed, when chest pain occurs. Nitrates are also available in a transdermal patch.

Tell 'em about tolerance

A patient can develop tolerance to nitroglycerin, regardless of the route of administration. Tolerance develops as the body becomes used to the effect of the drug; higher doses are then necessary to obtain the same effect. With all nitrates administered on a routine basis, a nitrate-free period is necessary every day to avoid tolerance.

Aspirin

Aspirin is a mild anticoagulant. By inhibiting platelet aggregation at the site of an obstruction, it may improve blood flow to the heart.

Second, yes; first, maybe

Because of its anticoagulant properties, aspirin can be taken daily (75 to 325 mg) to prevent a second heart attack. People who have taken aspirin regularly tend to have lower mortality rates if a second MI occurs.

The use of daily aspirin to prevent a first MI, however, hasn't been clinically proven. The patient should consult with his primary care provider about whether to use aspirin for primary prevention.

Beta-adrenergic blockers

Beta-adrenergic blockers are a required treatment after an MI, but many doctors also use them to help prevent MI in patients with angina. Beta-adrenergic blockers help to reduce the work of the heart by decreasing the heart rate.

Beta-adrenergic blockers work by blocking beta-adrenergic receptors in the heart. This decreases the number of stimuli the heart receives, thus decreasing heart rate, myocardial oxygen demand, and the number of angina attacks.

Common beta-adrenergic blockers include carvedilol (Coreg), propranolol (Inderal), metoprolol (Lopressor), atenolol (Tenormin), timolol (Blocadren), and nadolol (Corgard).

Quick quiz

1. A woman is more likely to suffer an MI:
- A. before menopause.
- B. after menopause.
- C. after age 45.

Answer: B. A woman is most likely to suffer an MI after menopause. Until then, estrogen helps protect her heart.

2. Nicotine use causes:
- A. the intima of an artery to become smooth.
- B. coronary vasodilation.
- C. coronary vasoconstriction.

Answer: C. Nicotine roughens and narrows the intima of the artery and leads to vasoconstriction.

3. Patients with diabetes are at risk for:
- A. silent MI.
- B. anterior MI.
- C. posterior MI.

Answer: A. Because of nerve damage, patients with diabetes are at risk for silent MI.

4. Aspirin helps prevent MI by:
   A. reducing preload.
   B. decreasing heart rate.
   C. inhibiting platelet aggregation.
Answer: C. Aspirin helps prevent MI by inhibiting platelet aggregation.

Scoring

☆☆☆ If you answered all four questions correctly, delightful! No modifications necessary for your study habits.

☆☆ If you answered three questions correctly, terrific! You've taken prevention to heart.

☆ If you answered fewer than three questions correctly, relax. There's no added risk to reading the chapter again.

3

Assessing patients with MI

> ### Key facts
> ◆ A key symptom of a myocardial infarction (MI) is crushing substernal chest pain.
> ◆ Women tend to experience different early signs of an MI than men do.
> ◆ When assessing the characteristics of a patient's MI pain, ask questions about type of pain, location, duration, radiation, precipitating events, and relieving factors.
> ◆ An electrocardiogram (ECG), one of the confirming tests for an MI, may reveal three pathological changes: infarction, injury, or ischemia.
> ◆ Cardiac enzyme level is another confirming test for an MI. Serum protein troponin level offers a new way to determine the presence of an MI.

Classic symptoms

The cardinal symptom of an MI is crushing, substernal pain that may radiate to the left arm, jaw, or shoulder blades. The pain may accompany nausea, vomiting,

Now I get it!

Angina or an MI?

Use the following guidelines to help distinguish pain caused by angina from pain that signals an MI.

Angina pain characteristics	MI pain characteristics
Occurs with exertion (physical or emotional)	Can occur at rest
Is relieved by rest	Isn't relieved by rest
Is relieved by nitroglycerin	Is relieved by morphine, rather than nitroglycerin
Lasts for minutes	Lasts for at least 20 minutes

diaphoresis, or dyspnea. An MI, unlike angina, can cause persistent pain for 12 hours or more. (See *Angina or an MI?*)

Also expect...

A patient experiencing an MI may report:
- a feeling of impending doom
- left-sided chest pain
- midscapular pain
- pain radiating down the right arm.

Cherchez la femme

Be aware that women tend to experience different early signs during MI than men. Learn to recognize these signs so that you can intervene effectively. (See *Recognizing MI in female patients,* page 40.)

Taking a history

The extent of your history will depend upon the patient's condition. If you suspect that the patient is experiencing an MI, only ask questions that will help guide your immediate plan of treatment. Remember that family members or anyone accompanying the patient may be a source of valuable information.

Information from your history may help you determine the origin of chest pain, or differentiate anginal pain from MI pain.

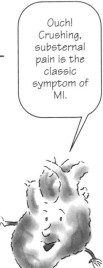

Ouch! Crushing, substernal pain is the classic symptom of MI.

Chief complaint

Ask why the patient is seeking medical treatment. Expect to hear a range of explanations, including:

• indigestion (long-lasting)

Advice from the experts

Recognizing MI in female patients

Though women may demonstrate the same symptoms as men during an MI, most experience different early symptoms. Typically, women don't experience the classic symptoms of MI until 1 hour into the MI. Until then, they generally experience vague complaints such as a sore neck and numbness and tingling in their right arm and hand.

- weakness
- dizziness
- difficulty breathing
- chest pain (mild or severe).

What's going on?

Ask questions about:

• *type of pain.* An MI usually causes a heavy-pressure, crushing, or squeezing pain, unaffected by changes in body position or respiration.

• *location.* Suspect an MI if the patient complains of substernal pain or radiating pain to the arm, neck, jaw, or back.

• *duration.* Sudden onset and pain that's continuous and prolonged suggests an MI.

Memory jogger

To remember key factors for assessing characteristics of a patient's chest pain, don't flip your lid, instead think *LID*:

Location **I**ntensity **D**uration.

• *precipitating events.* Stress, anxiety, exertion, temperature changes, and overeating typically bring on MI pain.
• *relieving factors.* Rest and nitroglycerin usually don't relieve MI pain immediately.

Medical history

Before attributing symptoms to an MI, ask the patient about:
• allergies to food, drugs, or other things
• use of prescription, over-the-counter, or recreational drugs.

If the situation isn't urgent, ask about cardiovascular risk factors:
• coronary artery disease
• diabetes
• high cholesterol
• hypertension
• previous cardiac events

- sedentary lifestyle
- smoking.

Also ask about past acute or chronic illnesses requiring hospitalization.

Family history

Ask if any blood relatives have had:
- cerebrovascular accidents
- diabetes
- heart disease
- hypertension
- renal disease.

Social history

After the patient's chest pain is relieved, ask about lifestyle, including:
- alcohol use
- diet
- exercise
- smoking.

Physical examination

A thorough physical examination is necessary to assess the patient for complications. Patients in critical condition — such as those in ventricular tachycardia, ventricular fibrillation, or cardiogenic

shock — require a thorough but rapid examination while interventions are performed. Techniques include:
• inspection
• percussion
• palpation
• auscultation.

Inspection

Look for evidence of MI, such as:
• ashen, or gray, skin color
• diaphoresis
• increased respiratory rate
• anxiety or restlessness
• jugular vein distention. (Distention is a sign of right ventricular infarction or heart failure.)

Percussion

Although percussion isn't as useful as other methods of assessment, the technique may help you locate cardiac borders.

Percuss the chest, noting any dullness. Begin percussing at the anterior axillary line. Percuss toward the sternum, along the fifth intercostal space. The sound changes from resonance to dullness over the left sternal border of the heart.

Palpation

Besides checking the standard pulse rate, which may be rapid, irregular, or slow, palpate the carotid pulse and the precordial pulse.

Gently palpate the carotid arteries, one side at a time. Palpating both at once can trigger severe bradycardia. The carotid artery is located in the groove between the trachea and the sternocleidomastoid muscle in the neck. Suspect reduced stroke volume if the pulse rate is hard to detect.

Also palpate for precordial pulsations. The pulsations occur during systole in patients with left ventricular dysfunction due to ischemic heart disease or a recent MI. In some patients, these abnormal pulsations may only be present during episodes of anginal pain. They're commonly felt in the midpericordium near the left ventricular apex.

Over each valve

Remember to palpate over each valve area. Perform both palpation and auscultation in the same sequence. (See *Sites for heart sounds,* page 45.)

Peak technique

Sites for heart sounds

Palpate and auscultate over each valve area:
- **aortic area:** second intercostal space, on the right sternal border
- **pulmonic area:** second intercostal space, on the left sternal border
- **second pulmonic area:** third intercostal space, on the left sternal border
- **tricuspid area:** fourth and fifth intercostal space, on the left sternal border
- **mitral area** (also called the apex): sixth intercostal space, on the midclavicular line.

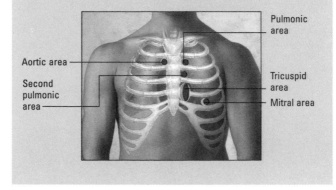

Palpation over the heart valves may detect a thrill. Presence of a thrill may indicate valvular problems or a ruptured papillary muscle (a complication of MI).

Auscultation

Auscultate the patient for heart sounds in three positions:

☝ lying on his back with the head of the bed raised 30 to 45 degrees

✌ lying on his left side

🖖 sitting up (See *Lub, dub, gallop, gallop.*)

The meaning of a murmur

When auscultating the patient, listen for a new onset murmur that may indicate a papillary muscle rupture. The most common valve affected by an MI is the mitral

Memory jogger

Use evolution to help remember valve order during palpation and auscultation. Think **AP**e **To Ma**n:

Aortic

Pulmonic

Tricuspid

Mitral.

Lub, dub, gallop, gallop

Here is a quick guide to four key heart sounds.

One, two

The first and second heart sounds (S_1 and S_2) are normal.

S_1 indicates closure of the atrioventricular valves and sounds like the word *lub*.

S_2 indicates closure of the semilunar valves and sounds like the word *dub*.

Three, four

The third and fourth heart sounds (S_3 and S_4), called gallop murmurs, are signs of fluid overload in adults.

S_3 occurs just after S_2 and may be caused by overdistention of the ventricles, mitral insufficiency, or heart failure.

S_4 occurs just before S_1 and indicates passive atrial filling. It may result from left ventricular hypertrophy, coronary artery disease, or aortic stenosis.

valve. Murmur may also indicate a rupture of the interventricular septum.

A drop

Auscultate the patient for blood pressure, which may drop from decreased cardiac output, increased vagal tone, or pain.

Diagnostic tests

Tests used to confirm a diagnosis of MI include electrocardiogram (ECG) testing and measurement of cardiac enzyme and serum protein troponin levels.

Tests used to assess damage caused by an MI include a cardiac catheterization, an echocardiogram, and radionuclide scan.

Electrocardiogram

When a patient enters an emergency unit, he is placed on a single- or dual-lead ECG. ECG monitoring may help detect arrhythmias, a common complication of MI. Depending on the lead, you may or may not see ECG changes. If ECG changes are present, you'll probably be able to note ST-segment elevation, a classic sign of MI.

To confirm an MI, a 12-lead ECG may be performed. A 12-lead ECG records information from 12 views of the heart, providing a complete picture of electrical activity. These 12 views are obtained by placing electrodes on the patient's limbs and chest. (See *Preparing the patient for a 12-lead ECG*.)

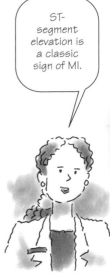

ST-segment elevation is a classic sign of MI.

Peak technique

Preparing the patient for a 12-lead ECG

Remind the patient that this procedure won't cause any pain. Make sure the patient lies completely still. Place the four limb leads in the correct places on the patient's extremities:

• **RL** goes on the right leg, on the inside part of the calf, midway between the knee and the ankle.
• **LL** goes on the left leg, on the inside part of the calf, midway between the knee and the ankle.
• **RA** goes on the right arm, inside, midway between the elbow and the shoulder.
• **LA** goes on the left arm, inside, midway between the elbow and the shoulder.

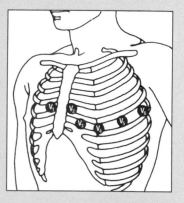

Chest leads

Place the six chest leads as shown in the illustration above.

• V_1: Fourth intercostal space, right sternal border

• V_2: Fourth intercostal space, left sternal border

• V_3: Halfway between V_2 and V_4

• V_4: Fifth intercostal space, mid-clavicular line

• V_5: Fifth intercostal space, anterior axillary line

• V_6: Fifth intercostal space, midaxillary line

Distinguishing type of injury

The zones of tissue damage in early acute MI include ischemia, injury, and infarction (also known as myocardial necrosis). An ECG may help to distinguish between ischemia, injury, and infarction. (See *Distinguishing types of tissue damage.*)

Pinpointing damage in the heart wall

Information from a 12-lead ECG can be used to detect specific sites of damage within the heart wall. Characteristic ECG changes that occur with an MI are localized to the leads overlying the infarction site. (See *Pinpointing an MI,* page 52.)

Important information may also be obtained by looking at the leads opposite the damaged area. These leads may reveal reciprocal ECG changes, which occur in the area of the heart opposite the MI. (See *Understanding reciprocal ECG changes,* page 53.)

Assessing right ventricular infarction

Most commonly an MI occurs in the left ventricle. However, a patient can develop an MI in the right ventricle or both ven-

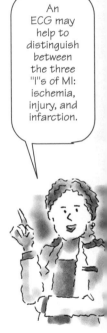

An ECG may help to distinguish between the three "I"s of MI: ischemia, injury, and infarction.

(Text continues on page 54.)

Peak technique

Distinguishing types of tissue damage

An ECG reading may help to distinguish types of tissue damage in an early acute MI.

Ischemia

In ischemia, an interrupted blood supply causes damage in the outermost area of the myocardium. Ischemia is represented on the ECG by T-wave inversion, as shown in the first strip below.

Injury

A prolonged lack of blood supply leads to myocardial injury. Injury is represented on the ECG by ST-segment elevation, as shown in the second strip below.

Infarction

This is the area of myocardial necrosis. Eventually, scar tissue replaces dead tissue. On an ECG strip, infarction is represented by a permanently pathological Q wave, indicating a lack of depolarization. Note that some MIs don't produce Q waves. These are known as non–Q wave MIs. In such MIs, damage doesn't involve all layers of the heart.

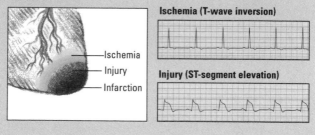

Ischemia

Injury

Infarction

Ischemia (T-wave inversion)

Injury (ST-segment elevation)

Peak technique

Pinpointing an MI

Information from a 12-lead ECG can be used to detect specific sites of damage in the heart wall. The chart below lists sites of heart wall damage, associated leads for characteristic ECG changes, and associated leads for reciprocal changes.

Note that a standard 12-lead ECG doesn't directly access the posterior wall. Therefore, in a standard 12-lead ECG, a posterior-wall MI can only be assessed through characteristic reciprocal changes in leads V_1 and V_2 (R wave greater than S wave; depressed ST segments; elevated T wave). A posterior ECG (with leads placed on the patient's back) may be performed to detect pathologic Q waves in leads V_7 through V_9.

Site of myocardial damage	Leads showing characteristic ECG changes	Leads showing reciprocal changes
Inferior wall	II, III, aV_F	aV_L
Lateral wall	I, aV_L, V_5, V_6	V_1, V_2
Anterior wall	V_2 to V_4	II, III, aV_F
Posterior wall	None	V_1, V_2
Anterolateral wall	I, aV_L, V_4 to V_6	II, II, aV_F
Anteroseptal wall	V_1 to V_3	None

Now I get it!

Understanding reciprocal ECG changes

On the right of the illustration below, you'll find characteristic ECG changes produced by leads that directly record electrical activity in damaged areas of the heart. On the left of the illustration, however, you'll find reciprocal changes. These changes are produced by leads recording electrical activity in the area of the heart opposite the area of infarction, ischemia, or injury.

For example, a lead that directly shows myocardial injury may produce ST-segment elevation on a waveform. However, another lead may show the reciprocal — or opposite — change, namely ST-segment depression.

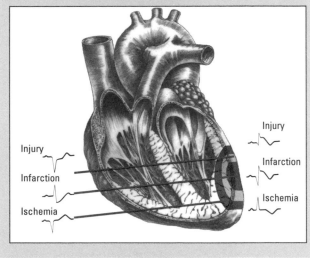

Injury

Infarction

Ischemia

Injury

Infarction

Ischemia

tricles. A right ventricular infarction usually occurs due to an occlusion of the right coronary artery.

A right ventricular infarction may be detected by performing an ECG on the right side of the heart. This means placing the precordial leads in a mirror image to a standard ECG. Look for classic ECG changes in precordial leads V_2R through V_6R:
• ST-segment elevation
• inverted T waves
• pathologic Q waves. (See *Assessing a patient for right ventricular infarction*.)

Cardiac enzyme level

Between 30 and 60 minutes after irreversible injury to myocardial tissue, certain enzymes and their isoenzymes spill into the plasma. To determine the presence of such enzymes, serial blood levels are performed every 6 to 8 hours for the first 24 hours of an MI and then daily.

High for 72 hours

Findings indicating an MI include elevated creatine kinase (CK) and myoglobin levels.

Peak technique

Assessing a patient for right ventricular infarction

Health care providers may overlook this type of infarction. To assess a patient for right ventricular infarction, check signs and symptoms discussed below.

Jugular vein distention
Right ventricular infarction causes blood to pool in the right ventricle, increasing filling pressure, leading to jugular vein distention.

Kussmaul's sign
Does inhalation accentuate jugular vein distention?

Clear lungs
Blood backs up on the heart's right side, so less blood reaches the lungs and congestion can't develop.

Hypotension
The left ventricle receives less blood, causing cardiac output to drop.

Heart block
The right coronary artery supplies blood to the atrioventricular node. An interruption in blood flow may cause varying degrees of heart block.

Abnormal heart sounds
The abnormal, third heart sound results from overdistention of the ventricles.

CK levels rise 4 to 8 hours after an MI. They tend to peak after 18 to 24 hours and stay high for up to 72 hours. To confirm an MI, 10% of the total enzymes must be CK-MB (an isoenzyme found in the heart).

Myoglobin levels rise 1 to 3 hours after an MI. They tend to peak at 4 hours and return to normal within 12 to 24 hours. Performing serial measurements of myoglobin levels increases test specificity and sensitivity. These levels are most helpful when used in conjunction with other cardiac markers, such as CK and troponin.

Serum protein troponin level

Measurement of a cardiac protein called troponin offers the most precise way to determine if a patient has experienced an MI. Some 6 hours after the MI, a blood test can detect two forms of troponin: T and I. Levels of Troponin T peak about 2 days after an MI and return to normal range about 16 days after an MI. Levels of Troponin I reach their peak in less than a day after an MI and return to normal range in about 7 days.

Detection of either form of troponin provides conclusive evidence of an MI. Higher troponin levels have been associated with an increased risk of mortality.

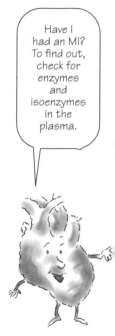

Have I had an MI? To find out, check for enzymes and isoenzymes in the plasma.

Cardiac catheterization

Cardiac catheterization is used to study the heart, large blood vessels, and coronary arteries and to determine the presence and extent of coronary artery disease. For patients with an acute MI, this test may be performed as an adjunct to an angioplasty.

Radionuclide scan

A radionuclide scan helps to measure heart function and damage. During this test, a mildly radioactive element is injected into the patient's bloodstream. Computer-generated pictures are used to locate the mildly radioactive element in the heart. This test takes 1½ to 2 hours. Results from the test help to determine:

• how well the heart muscle is supplied with blood

• how well the heart chambers are functioning

• which part of the heart was damaged by the MI

• how much damage the MI has caused to the heart muscle.

In a technetium scan of the heart, the technician injects the patient with technetium 99, a mildly radioactive substance. Damaged areas of the myocardium show up as "hot spots" on the film.

In a thallium scan, the patient is injected with a mildly radioactive substance called thallium 201. Poorly perfused areas and coronary spasms show up as "cold spots" on the film.

Transthoracic echocardiogram

Transthoracic echocardiogram is a noninvasive test that's used to examine the size, shape, and motion of cardiac structures. In a patient with an MI, an echocardiogram may be performed to evaluate motion of the heart wall.

In an echocardiogram, a special transducer placed at an acoustic window on the patient's chest (an area where bone and lung tissue are absent) directs ultrahigh frequency sound waves to cardiac structures. Cardiac structures reflect these waves back. The echoes of these sound waves are converted by oscilloscope for display on a monitor, strip chart, or videotape.

Quick quiz

1. When doing a 12-lead ECG, lead V_4 is placed at the:

    A. fourth intercostal space, left sternal border.

    B. fourth intercostal space, right sternal border.

    C. fifth intercostal space, midclavicular line.

Answer: C. V_4 is placed in the fifth intercostal space of the midclavicular line.

2. The leads that look at the inferior wall of the heart are:

    A. II, III, aV_F.

    B. I, aV_L, V_5, V_6.

    C. I, aV_L, V_4, V_6.

Answer: A. The inferior leads are II, III, and aV_F.

3. A cardiac catheterization may be performed with:

    A. a stress test.

    B. a radionuclide scan.

    C. an angioplasty.

Answer: C. Cardiac catheterization is done in conjunction with an angioplasty to open a blocked artery.

4. The classic symptom of an MI is:

A.   jaw pain.

B.   back pain.

C.   substernal pain.

Answer: C. Classic MI pain is described as crushing substernal pain. However, these other types of pain can also indicate MI.

Scoring

☆☆☆   If you answered three or four questions correctly, excellent! Your expertise in ECGs is electrifying.

☆☆   If you answered fewer than three questions correctly, don't fret. It takes more than one test to confirm a diagnosis, and there are three more quick quizzes to go.

4

Treating patients with MI

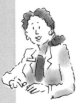

Key facts

- ◆ During an acute MI, thrombolytics are used to dissolve a thrombus in the coronary artery and reperfuse the myocardium.
- ◆ Beta-adrenergic blockers are standard of care medications for post-myocardial infarction (MI) patients.
- ◆ In percutaneous transluminal coronary angioplasty, a balloon-tipped catheter is used to open blocked coronary arteries.
- ◆ A stent — a metal, springlike device — is placed into a narrowed coronary artery to hold it open permanently.
- ◆ In a coronary artery bypass graft, the most common surgery used to treat an MI, a grafted vessel is used to divert blood flow around a blocked coronary artery.

Treating MI with drugs

Immediately after an MI, your patient needs specific drugs, such as aspirin and a thrombolytic, to restore blood flow to

Initial MI treatment goals
• Reduce pain.
• Prevent further myocardial damage.
• Increase tissue oxygenation.
• Decrease myocardial oxygen consumption.
• Maintain adequate cardiac output.

the heart. (See *Initial MI treatment goals*.)

The patient also needs supplemental oxygen for at least the first 24 to 48 hours after the MI. Oxygen therapy helps keep the heart and other tissues well oxygenated.

After the initial treatment period, the patient needs further drug therapy to help regulate cardiovascular function and prevent complications.

Aspirin

Aspirin is a blood thinner that reduces platelet aggregation, improving blood flow through the coronary arteries and into the heart.

Right now

A patient should take an aspirin as soon as he realizes he is having an MI. If he hasn't taken one by the time he reaches the emergency room, he should receive one immediately.

Thrombolytic agents

During an acute MI, thrombolytics are used to dissolve a thrombus in the coronary artery and reperfuse the stunned myocardium. When reperfusion occurs, the myocardium receives oxygen-rich blood. (See *Common thrombolytics,* pages 64 and 65.)

The window shuts quickly

Thrombolytic therapy should start within 4 to 6 hours after the symptoms begin. After the 4-to-6-hour window, the benefits and chance of successful reperfusion decrease, although beneficial effects may extend for up to 12 hours and possibly longer.

Before...

Obtain a thorough patient history and double-check when chest pain began.

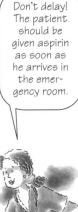

Don't delay! The patient should be given aspirin as soon as he arrives in the emergency room.

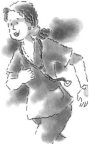

(Text continues on page 66.)

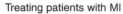

Common thrombolytics

alteplase (recombinant tissue plasminogen activator [rt-PA])
Trade name: Activase

Indications
Lysis of thrombi obstructing coronary arteries during acute MI

Adverse effects
Cerebral hemorrhage; arrhythmia; severe, spontaneous bleeding; hypersensitivity reactions

Special considerations
Don't exceed 100 mg/dose. Higher doses are associated with an increased incidence of intracranial bleeding.

anistreplase (anisoylated plasminogen-streptokinase activator complex [APSAC])
Trade name: Eminase

Indications
Lysis of thrombi obstructing coronary arteries during acute MI

Adverse effects
Intracranial hemorrhage, arrhythmia, bleeding, anaphylaxis or anaphylactoid reactions

Special considerations
Give anistreplase by I.V. push because it's activated slowly in the bloodstream.

reteplase, recombinant (recombinant plasminogen activator, rPA)
Trade name: Retavase

Indications
Management of acute MI, lysis of coronary artery thrombi

Common thrombolytics *(continued)*

Adverse effects
Intracranial hemorrhage, arrhythmia, cholesterol embolization, hemorrhage

Special considerations
Monitor electrocardiogram; be prepared to treat bradycardia or ventricular irritability; avoid I.M. injections, invasive procedures, and nonessential handling of patient.

---

streptokinase
Trade name: Streptase

Indications
Lysis of thrombi obstructing coronary arteries during acute MI

Adverse effects
Hypotension and allergic reactions, reperfusion arrhythmias, bleeding, bronchospasm, pulmonary edema, urticaria, flushing

Special considerations
If allergic reaction occurs but responds to treatment, don't discontinue drug.

---

urokinase
Trade name: Abbokinase

Indications
Lysis of thrombi obstructing coronary arteries during acute MI

Adverse effects
Hypotension, reperfusion arrhythmias, bleeding, bronchospasm, fever, chills, nausea, hypersensitivity reaction

Special considerations
Before giving urokinase, give 2,500 to 10,000 U of heparin by rapid I.V. injection.

Also establish all necessary I.V. sites and include a spare heparin lock for later use.

...during...

During thrombolytic therapy, prepare and administer the medication as prescribed. Monitor the patient's electrocardiogram (ECG) for transient arrhythmias, and remember to flush the system when the infusion is complete to ensure that the patient receives all the medication.

Thrombolysis typically occurs 30 to 45 minutes after therapy starts. When this occurs, chest pain resolves. Creatine kinase levels peak up to 12 hours after therapy begins.

...after

Monitor the patient for:
• arrhythmias
• bleeding
• diaphoresis
• nausea
• recurrence of chest pain
• ST-segment elevation.

Heparin

Depending on the drug administered, patients who receive thrombolytic therapy may receive I.V. heparin to facilitate thrombolysis. Immediate administration of heparin after administration of clot-specific thrombolytic drugs, such as alteplase and reteplase, diminishes reocclusion after successful reperfusion. Scant evidence exists supporting the use of I.V. heparin in patients who don't receive thrombolytic therapy.

If not contraindicated, heparin may be administered subcutaneously to patients who haven't received thrombolytic therapy.

I may deliver heparin to patients who receive clot-specific thrombolytic agents.

Additional blood thinning drugs

Aspirin may be administered along with thrombolytic therapy to help prevent newly dissolved clots from clotting again in the patient's blood vessels.

After the critical period has passed, other blood thinning drugs (for example, warfarin, ticlopidine, and enoxaparin) may be administered. Teach the patient to monitor for bleeding by watching his urine for blood clots, noting any nasal bleeding, and observing for rectal bleeding.

Long-term therapy

To help prevent future episodes of MI, the primary care provider may prescribe long-term therapy with up to 325 mg (one tablet) of aspirin per day. Patients who receive long-term aspirin therapy should watch for petechiae, bleeding gums, and signs of GI bleeding, such as blood-streaked stool or vomitus.

Beta-adrenergic blockers

Beta blockers are considered the standard of care right after an MI. These drugs reduce stress on the myocardium by slowing the heart rate and decreasing the strength of the heart's contractions.

Beta blockers can prevent some MI patients from developing serious ventricular arrhythmias. They may also be used in long-term therapy for their antihypertensive effects. These drugs vary slightly in the way they work, but all tend to produce similar adverse reactions. (See *Common beta blockers*.)

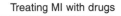

Common beta blockers

atenolol
Trade name: Tenormin

Indications
To reduce mortality and risk of reinfarction in patients with acute MI

Adverse effects
Fatigue, lethargy, vertigo, dizziness, bradycardia, heart failure, hypotension, nausea, diarrhea, bronchospasm, dyspnea

Special considerations
Use cautiously in patients at risk for heart failure and in those with bronchospastic disease, diabetes mellitus, and hyperthyroidism; withhold from patients with pulse lower than 60 beats/minute; if administering I.V., don't exceed 1 mg/minute; I.V. doses may be mixed with dextrose 5% in water, normal saline solution, or dextrose and normal saline solutions; solution is stable for 48 hours after mixing; monitor blood pressure; withdraw gradually over 2 weeks to avoid serious adverse effects.

metoprolol tartrate
Trade name: Lopressor

Indications
To reduce mortality after MI and improve myocardial supply-demand relationship

Adverse effects
Fatigue, lethargy, dizziness, bradycardia, hypotension, heart failure, nausea, vomiting, diarrhea, dyspnea, bronchospasm, rash, fever, arthralgia, impotence

(continued)

Common beta blockers *(continued)*

Special considerations
Use cautiously in patients with heart failure, diabetes, or respiratory or hepatic disease; withhold from patients with pulse lower than 60 beats/minute; if given I.V., administer undiluted and avoid mixing with other drugs; monitor blood glucose in diabetic patients; monitor blood pressure frequently.

---

propranolol hydrochloride
Trade name: Inderal

Indications
To reduce mortality after MI

Adverse effects
Fatigue, lethargy, vivid dreams, bradycardia, hypotension, heart failure, peripheral vascular disease, nausea, vomiting, diarrhea, dyspnea, bronchospasm, increased airway resistance, rash, fever, impotence

Special considerations
Use cautiously in patients with renal impairment, diabetes mellitus, nonallergic bronchospastic diseases, or hepatic diseases; check pulse and withhold from patients with extremes in pulse rate; if administering I.V., use a large vessel or tubing of free-flowing, compatible I.V. solution; avoid continuous I.V. infusion ; if administering by mouth, give consistently with meals; monitor blood pressure, electrocardiogram, and heart rate and rhythm frequently, especially during I.V. infusion.

Nitrates

Nitrates are used to treat angina and acute MI. Nitrates decrease the heart's workload by:

• reducing the amount of blood that returns to the heart

• decreasing blood pressure and reducing the force the left ventricle must exert to pump the blood

• dilating the coronary arteries, which increases the blood supply to the myocardium, thereby relieving the pain associated with an MI.

Nitrates reduce my workload.

Know your nitrates

Nitrates may be given by the I.V., transdermal, or sublingual route. Typically, the I.V. route is used for short-term therapy and the other routes are used for long-term therapy.

Oh no! Dizziness, weakness, hypotension...

Watch for adverse reactions, including headache (sometimes throbbing), dizziness, weakness, orthostatic hypotension, tachycardia, flushing, palpitations, fainting, nausea, vomiting, rash, and sublingual burning. Administer nitrates cautiously to a patient with hypotension or volume depletion because these drugs can quickly reduce blood pressure.

ACE inhibitors

Angiotensin-converting enzyme (ACE) inhibitors block the conversion of angiotensin I (a weak vasoconstrictor) to angiotensin II (a potent vasoconstrictor). This action lessens afterload demand (the force the left ventricle must overcome to eject blood into the systemic circulation) during an MI. ACE inhibitors have been shown to preserve left ventricular function and reduce the rate of mortality for MI patients. (See *Common ACE inhibitors.*)

Help for high-risk

ACE inhibitors provide the most benefit for high-risk patients such as:
- the elderly
- those who have suffered an anterior MI
- those who have experienced a previous MI
- those with depressed left ventricular function.

Look out for low pressure

Because ACE inhibitors lower blood pressure, they should be used cautiously if the patient has a systolic blood pressure less than 100 mm Hg.

Common ACE inhibitors

captopril
Trade name: Captoten

Indications
To reduce mortality and slow the development of heart failure post-MI

Adverse effects
Leukopenia; thrombocytopenia; agranulocytosis; dry, persistent, nonproductive cough; urticarial rash; maculopapular rash; hypotension; tachycardia

Special considerations
Use cautiously in patients with impaired renal function or serious autoimmune disease (such as systemic lupus erythematosus) or in patients taking drugs that affect white blood cell (WBC) count or immune response; monitor patient's blood pressure and pulse rate frequently; be aware that elderly patients may be more sensitive to drug's hypotensive effects.

enalapril maleate
Trade name: Vasotec

Indications
To control hypertension

Adverse effects
Dizziness; headache; fatigue; vertigo; hypotension; dry, persistent, nonproductive cough; neutropenia; thrombocytopenia; agranulocytosis

Special considerations
Use cautiously in patients with impaired renal function; monitor blood pressure response closely; monitor complete blood count with differential counts before and during therapy.

(continued)

Common ACE inhibitors *(continued)*

lisinopril
Trade name: Prinivil

Indications
To reduce mortality after MI

Adverse effects
Agranulocytosis; dry, persistent, nonproductive cough; dizziness; headache; fatigue; hypotension

Special considerations
Use cautiously in patients with impaired renal function; monitor blood pressure often; monitor WBC with differential counts before therapy, every 2 weeks for first 3 months of therapy, and periodically thereafter; because angioedema can occur, teach patient to recognize and report swelling or breathing difficulty.

Treatment using ACE inhibitors should generally start within the first 24 hours after an MI — after thrombolytic therapy is complete and the patient's blood pressure is stable.

Morphine

Morphine is the drug of choice for treating MI pain during the acute period. Morphine binds with opiate receptors in the central nervous system, altering the patient's perception of — and emotional response to — pain through an unknown mechanism.

The right route

Morphine is most effective when administered by the I.V. route. When given by injection, it may lead to false elevations in enzyme studies.

Morphine is usually given in small doses (2 to 4 mg) and may be administered as often as every 5 minutes as tolerated.

Respiratory check

Because morphine acts as a sedative, make sure the patient's respiratory function is adequate before starting this drug.

During administration, monitor the patient's blood pressure because morphine can increase hypotension. Also monitor the patient closely for signs of cardiopulmonary distress, such as bradycardia, bradypnea, and apnea.

Morphine is most effective when administered by the I.V. route.

Antiarrhythmics

Antiarrhythmics help regulate the
rhythm of the heart after an MI. They're
used to treat the ventricular arrhythmias
that may result from an MI, such as sus-
tained ventricular tachycardia and ventricular fibrillation. (See *Common antiarrhythmics*.)

Adrenergics

Adrenergics directly stimulate the
heart's beta receptors to increase myocardial contractility and stroke volume,
thereby increasing cardiac output.

Adrenergics are given directly after
an MI to compensate for the damaged
ventricle's inability to contract. Dobutamine hydrochloride (Dobutrex) and
dopamine hydrochloride (Intropin)
are common adrenergics.

Central or peripheral

Administer adrenergics by I.V., using a
central venous catheter or large peripheral vein. Titrate the dosage based on the
patient's condition.

During adrenergic therapy, monitor the
patient's ECG, blood pressure, and urine

> Adrenergics directly stimulate my beta receptors to increase myocardial contractility and stroke volume.

Common antiarrhythmics

atropine sulfate
Trade name: None

Indications
Symptomatic bradycardia or bradyarrhythmia resulting from an MI

Adverse effects
Headache, restlessness, disorientation, coma, palpitations, tachycardia, angina, blurred vision, dry mouth, urine retention

Special considerations
Administer via direct I.V. into a large vein or I.V. tubing over at least 1 minute; monitor patient for paradoxical initial bradycardia; watch for tachycardia, which can lead to ventricular fibrillation.

lidocaine hydrochloride
Trade name: Xylocaine

Indications
Ventricular arrhythmia resulting from MI

Adverse effects
Confusion, tremor, lethargy, somnolence, seizures, hypotension, bradycardia, new or worsened arrhythmias, tinnitus, blurred vision, anaphylaxis

Special considerations
Use cautiously in patients with complete or second-degree heart block or with sinus bradycardia, in elderly patients, in those with heart failure or renal or hepatic disease; patients receiving infusions must be on a cardiac monitor; monitor patients for seizures or other signs of toxicity.

output. Also check for adverse reactions, such as headache, increased heart rate, hypertension, premature ventricular contractions, angina, nausea, vomiting, shortness of breath, and mild leg cramps.

Antianxiety drugs

Antianxiety drugs are commonly used to keep the patient calm during the acute phase of an MI as well as to help the patient sleep during the initial period in the coronary care unit. Common antianxiety drugs include diazepam (Valium), lorazepam (Ativan), and alprazolam (Xanax).

Monitor the patient for signs of oversedation, such as lethargy, bradycardia, and decreased respiration.

Diuretics

Diuretics may be given to a patient after an MI to relieve signs of fluid overload such as:
• jugular vein distention
• edema
• crackles
• positive hepatojugular reflex.

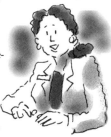

During the acute phase of an MI, antianxiety drugs are commonly used to keep the patient calm.

I.V. initially, oral later

Diuretics are often administered I.V. during the initial treatment of an MI. The patient may then switch to oral diuretics after he has stabilized.

Monitor the patient taking diuretics for signs of dehydration and hypokalemia.

Treating MI with procedures

In conjunction with medications, or in place of them, a doctor may order procedures such as:

• percutaneous transluminal coronary angioplasty (PTCA)
• placement of a coronary artery stent
• pulmonary artery pressure monitoring
• intra-aortic balloon counterpulsation (IABC)
• implantation of a ventricular assist device.

In addition, an experimental procedure called transmyocardial revascularization (TMR) provides an alternative for patients not eligible for coronary artery bypass graft (CABG) or PTCA. (See *Talking about TMR*, page 80.)

Battling illness

Talking about TMR

Transmyocardial revascularization (TMR) is a relatively new procedure that uses a carbon dioxide laser to cut a series of transmural channels in the heart's left ventricle. These channels then allow blood flow to ischemic heart tissue.

Percutaneous transluminal coronary angioplasty

In PTCA, a balloon-tipped catheter is used to open blocked coronary arteries. The balloon is inserted into the coronary artery and inflated where the artery narrows. There the balloon compresses plaque against the vessel wall, allowing coronary blood to flow more freely.

Effective but not without risks

Clinical studies show that PTCA offers better short-term and long-term outcomes than thrombolytic therapy. PTCA can cause complications, however. (See *PTCA: Potential problems.*)

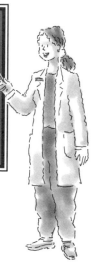

PTCA: Potential problems
- Coronary artery occlusion
- Coronary artery spasm
- Dissection of coronary artery
- Extension of MI
- Hematoma
- Hemorrhage
- Restenosis of the affected artery

Coronary stent

A stent is a metal, springlike device that is placed into a narrowed coronary artery to hold it open permanently.

When PTCA doesn't work

A stent is often used when PTCA has failed repeatedly. The patient usually must take an antiplatelet drug for 2 to 4 weeks after receiving a stent.

A stent can sometimes lead to adverse effects, such as:
- arrhythmias
- dissection of the coronary artery
- hematoma at the insertion site
- hemorrhage

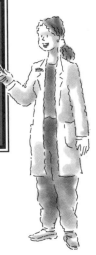

IABC complications
• Arterial embolism
• Extension or rupture of an aortic aneurysm
• Femoral perforation
• Femoral artery occlusion
• Sepsis
• Thrombocytopenia

• restenosis of the stented segment
• stent thrombosis or occlusion.

Pulmonary artery pressure monitoring

This procedure involves using a balloon-tipped catheter to measure pulmonary artery pressure, pulmonary artery wedge pressure, and cardiac output. The doctor can then use these measurements to assess damage caused by the MI and make decisions about treatment.

IABC

With IABC, a balloon-tipped catheter is inserted through the femoral artery into the descending thoracic aorta. The

IABC in action

Intra-aortic balloon counterpulsation (IABC) displaces blood in the aorta by means of a balloon attached to an external pump console. The illustrations here show the direction of blood flow when the pump inflates and deflates the balloon.

Balloon inflation   **Balloon deflation**

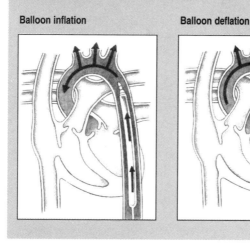

catheter is attached to an external pump, which inflates the balloon during diastole. This pushes blood through the aorta into the coronary arteries. (See *IABC complications* and *IABC in action*.) IABC reduces the heart's workload and is commonly used to treat patients with cardiogenic shock.

Stabilizing effect

Typically used as a temporary measure, IABC helps stabilize patients waiting for CABG surgery, as well as those with:
• cardiogenic shock after an MI
• significant hypotension
• uncontrolled chest pain.

Ventricular assist device

The ventricular assist device (VAD) is a temporary life-sustaining treatment for a failing heart. (See *Assisting a failing heart.*) It diverts systemic blood flow from a diseased ventricle into a centrifugal pump, which returns the blood to the circulation. This reduces the ventricle's workload and lets the myocardium rest.

> Replace me? A VAD can do it for a short time while I rest.

Like an artificial heart

The VAD functions like an artificial heart. It's implanted in the patient's chest cavity and receives power through the skin from an external belt of electrical transformer coils that work as a

Assisting a failing heart

Unlike an artificial heart, a ventricular assist device (VAD) helps the failing heart by assisting it rather than replacing it. The illustration here shows how the parts of the VAD work with the heart.

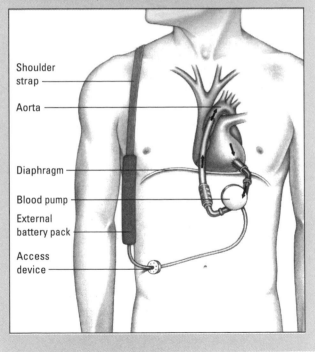

Shoulder strap

Aorta

Diaphragm

Blood pump

External battery pack

Access device

Battling illness

Two methods of CABG surgery

During coronary artery bypass graft (CABG) surgery, the surgeon may use several saphenous vein grafts or he may use a single internal mammary artery graft, as shown below.

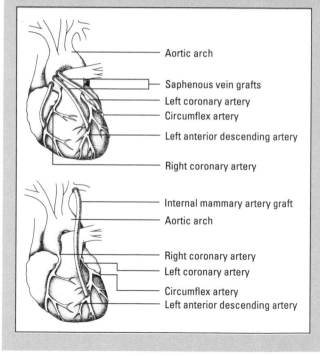

portable battery pack. The device can also operate off an implanted, recharge-able battery for up to 1 hour.

Complications may include cerebrovas-cular accident and pulmonary embolism.

Treating MI with surgery

If PTCA and other procedures aren't ef-fective, the patient may undergo CABG surgery.

Coronary artery bypass graft

In CABG surgery, a grafted vessel is used to divert blood flow around a blocked coronary artery. This provides oxygen to areas of the myocardium suf-fering from decreased blood supply, re-ducing angina and improving the pa-tient's quality of life.

For the grafted vessel, the surgeon uses a portion of a healthy vessel from another part of the body. (See *Two meth-ods of CABG surgery*.)

Quick quiz

1. The standard-of-care medications for post-MI patients are:

    A. nitrates.

    B. beta-adrenergic blockers.

    C. calcium channel blockers.

Answer: B. Beta-adrenergic blockers are the standard of care for post-MI patients.

2. Coronary artery bypass graft (CABG) surgery is performed to:

    A. prevent cerebrovascular accident.

    B. prevent another MI.

    C. decrease angina.

Answer: C. The primary purpose of CABG surgery is to decrease angina. In some cases it may also extend the patient's life.

Scoring

☆☆☆   If you answered both questions correctly, marvelous! You've eliminated all the blockages to knowledge.

☆☆   If you answered fewer than two questions correctly, no worries. Reading the chapter again offers a noninvasive way to improve.

5

MI complications

Key facts
- Arrhythmias, the most common complication of an MI, occur when the heart's normal electrical pathway becomes impaired.
- Cardiac arrest is the most common emergency complication of MI. During cardiac arrest, the patient's heart fails to produce a life-sustaining rhythm.
- Cardiogenic shock affects 10% to 20% of patients with acute MI. Without proper treatment, it can lead to death.
- Heart failure occurs when the heart can't pump enough blood to meet the body's metabolic needs. Heart failure accounts for one-third of all MI deaths.

Dangers after MI

Your patient's risk of complications depends on where the MI occurred, the amount of tissue necrosis, and the degree of function remaining in the left ventricle. (See *Post-MI complications,* page 90.)

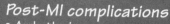

Post-MI complications
- Arrhythmias
- Cardiac arrest
- Cardiac muscle dysfunction
- Cardiogenic shock
- GI complications
- Heart failure
- Mitral insufficiency
- Pericarditis
- Thromboembolism

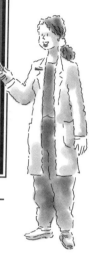

Arrhythmias

The most common complication of MI, arrhythmias occur when the heart's normal electrical pathway becomes impaired, causing the heart to beat in an altered way. (See *Common arrhythmias*.)

Atrial fibrillation

Atrial fibrillation (AF) is a transient arrhythmia that usually occurs within the first 24 hours after an acute MI. AF is marked by the absence of P waves and

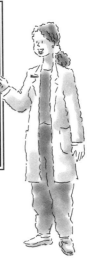

> ### Common arrhythmias
> • Atrial fibrillation
> • Premature ventricular contractions
> • Ventricular tachycardia
> • Accelerated idioventricular rhythm
> • Ventricular fibrillation
> • Atrioventricular heart block

by an irregular ventricular response. (See *Spotting atrial fibrillation*, page 92.)

Increased odds

The chance of AF increases with age. The condition occurs most commonly in patients with:
• anterior infarctions
• larger infarctions
• heart failure
• pericarditis.

Decreased risk

Thrombolytic therapy tends to decrease the incidence of AF.

Don't skip this strip

Spotting atrial fibrillation

This electrocardiogram strip shows atrial fibrillation. Note that the sinus P wave is replaced by erratic fibrillatory waves.

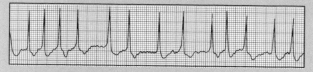

Also notice these distinguishing characteristics:
- *rhythm:* irregularly irregular
- *rate:* atrial, indiscernible; ventricular, 130 beats/minute
- *P wave:* absent; replaced by fine fibrillatory waves
- *PR interval:* indiscernible
- *QRS complex:* 0.08 second
- *T wave:* indiscernible
- *QT interval:* unmeasurable.

From A(F) to B(eta blocker)

AF is usually treated with a beta blocker such as atenolol or metoprolol. If the patient's condition fails to stabilize, he may need cardioversion.

Premature ventricular contractions

Although premature ventricular contractions (PVCs) may occur after any MI, they usually occur after an MI that damages the ventricles. On the patient's electrocardiogram (ECG) strip, PVCs appear as a single or coupled ventricular beat that occurs before the normal QRS complex. (See *Spotting PVCs,* page 94.)

Danger ahead

Certain PVCs are especially dangerous and may progress to ventricular tachycardia. (See *When PVCs signal danger,* pages 95 and 96.)

Treat with antiarrhythmics

Treating PVCs usually requires an antiarrhythmic, such as lidocaine and procainamide.

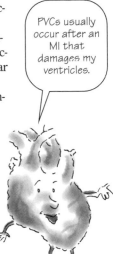

PVCs usually occur after an MI that damages my ventricles.

Ventricular tachycardia

Three or more consecutive PVCs constitute ventricular tachycardia. This arrhythmia can develop after any type of MI and may occur suddenly, cease suddenly, or occur continuously. Ventricular tachycardia increases the patient's risk of

Don't skip this strip

Spotting PVCs

This electrocardiogram strip shows premature ventricular contractions (PVCs) on beats 1, 6, and 11. Note the wide and bizarre appearance of the QRS complex.

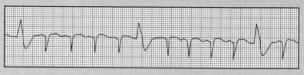

Also notice these distinguishing characteristics:
- *rhythm:* irregular
- *rate:* 120 beats/minute
- *P wave:* none with PVC, but P wave present with other QRS complexes
- *PR interval:* 0.12 second in underlying rhythm
- *QRS complex:* early, with bizarre configuration and duration of 0.14 second in PVC; normal QRS complexes are 0.08 second
- *T wave:* normal; opposite direction from QRS complex
- *QT interval:* 0.28 second in underlying rhythm.

sudden cardiac death. (See *Spotting ventricular tachycardia,* page 97.)

When PVCs signal danger

Here are some examples of patterns of dangerous premature ventricular contractions (PVCs).

Paired PVCs

Two PVCs in a row are called a pair or couplet (see highlighted areas). A pair can produce ventricular tachycardia because the second contraction usually meets refractory tissue. A salvo—three or more PVCs in a row—is considered a run of ventricular tachycardia.

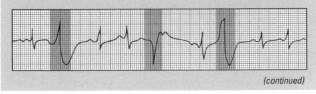

Multiform PVCs

PVCs that look different from one another arise from different sites or from the same site with abnormal conduction (see highlighted areas).

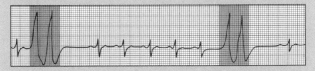

(continued)

When PVCs signal danger *(continued)*

Bigeminy and trigeminy

PVCs that occur every other beat (bigeminy) or every third beat (trigeminy) can result in ventricular tachycardia or ventricular fibrillation (see highlighted areas).

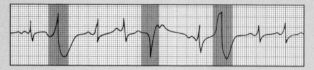

R-on-T phenomenon

In this phenomenon, the PVC occurs so early that it falls on the T wave of the preceding beat (see highlighted area). Because the cells haven't fully repolarized, ventricular tachycardia or ventricular fibrillation can result.

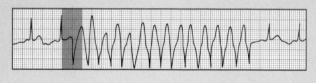

Treat with lidocaine, cardioversion, defibrillation

Treat this arrhythmia with lidocaine and, if the patient is unstable and the rhythm persists, cardioversion. If the patient develops recurrent ventricular tachycardia, he may be a candidate for an implantable

Spotting ventricular tachycardia

This electrocardiogram strip shows identifying characteristics of ventricular tachycardia.

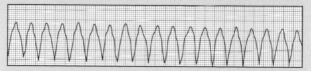

On this strip, you'll find the following characteristics:
- *rhythm:* regular
- *rate:* 187 beats/minute
- *P wave:* absent
- *PR interval:* not measurable
- *QRS complex:* 0.24 second; wide and bizarre
- *T wave:* opposite direction from QRS complex
- *QT interval:* not measurable.

cardiac defibrillator. (See *Inside action,* page 98.)

Accelerated idioventricular rhythm

Accelerated idioventricular rhythm usually develops as a result of reperfusion or after an inferior wall MI.

Battling illness

Inside action

An implantable cardiac defibrillator (ICD), which consists of one or more leads and a defibrillator unit, is implanted to help control ventricular tachycardia. The leads carry signals from the heart to the defibrillator, prompting a response when the tachycardia occurs. Implantation of an ICD uses similar methods to those of a permanent pacemaker.

Three in a row

In this arrhythmia, three or more successive ventricular beats occur at a rate of 60 to 100 beats/minute. The rhythm may begin with a long coupling interval with fusion beats at the beginning and end. (See *Spotting accelerated idioventricular rhythm,* page 100.)

Possibly a pacemaker

There's usually no treatment, although the patient may need a pacemaker if his heart rate is excessively slow or if he develops hypotension.

Ventricular fibrillation

Ventricular fibrillation occurs in two main forms:

👆 primary, which occurs most commonly in the first 4 hours after MI

✌️ late, which develops more than 48 hours after the MI and usually results from heart failure or cardiogenic shock.

On an ECG strip, this arrhythmia appears as electrical chaos with no discernible complexes. (See *Spotting ventricular fibrillation,* page 101.) It indicates that the heart isn't pumping.

Treat fibrillation with defibrillation

Defibrillation is necessary to treat ventricular fibrillation. As with ventricular tachycardia, any MI patient with ventricular fibrillation is at an increased risk for sudden death.

> Ouch. It's a shock but defibrillation will help me recover from ventricular fibrillation.

AV heart block

In atrioventricular (AV) heart block, the atria and the ventricles fail to work together properly. This arrhythmia usually

Don't skip this strip

Spotting accelerated idioventricular rhythm

This electrocardiogram strip shows an accelerated idioventricular rhythm.

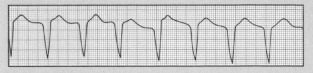

On this strip, you'll see the following distinguishing characteristics:
• *rhythm:* irregular
• *rate:* unable to determine atrial rate; ventricular rate of 60 to 100 beats/minute
• *P wave:* absent
• *PR interval:* not measurable
• *QRS complex:* 0.20 second and bizarre
• *T wave:* directly opposite last part of QRS complex
• *QT interval:* 0.46 second.

develops in patients who have suffered an acute MI. It occurs in three main forms:

first degree, in which the impulse from the atria to the ventricles is delayed

second degree, in which the impulse

Don't skip this strip

Spotting ventricular fibrillation

This electrocardiogram strip shows coarse ventricular fibrillation.

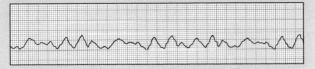

To interpret this strip, notice the following distinguishing characteristics:

- *rhythm:* chaotic
- *rate:* undetermined
- *P wave:* absent
- *PR interval:* not measurable
- *QRS complex:* indiscernible
- *T wave:* indiscernible
- *QT interval:* not applicable
- *other:* waveform is a wavy line.

is progressively delayed or intermittently not conducted

third degree, also known as complete heart block, in which communication between the atria and ventricles ceases and each beats on their own. (See *Spotting AV heart block,* page 102.)

Don't skip this strip

Spotting AV heart block

The following electrocardiogram strip shows third-degree atrioventricular (AV) heart block, also known as complete heart block.

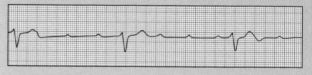

To interpret this strip, look for these distinguishing characteristics:
- *rhythm:* regular
- *rate:* atrial, 90 beats/minute; ventricular, 30 beats/minute
- *P wave:* normal
- *PR interval:* not measurable
- *QRS complex:* 0.16 second
- *T wave:* normal
- *QT interval:* 0.56 second.

Sometimes sudden, other times gradual

Complete heart block tends to occur suddenly in patients with anterior wall MI. It develops gradually in patients with inferior wall MI. Typically, it's treated with a pacemaker, though the patient may receive atropine while preparing for the pacemaker insertion.

Warning!

Arresting behavior

During cardiac arrest, a patient typically shows life-threatening signs, such as:
- no pulse
- no respirations
- unconsciousness
- ventricular fibrillation on electrocardiogram strip.

Cardiac arrest

Cardiac arrest is the most common emergency complication caused by an MI. During cardiac arrest, the patient's heart fails to produce a life-sustaining rhythm. (See *Arresting behavior.*)

Treat with defibrillation, epinephrine...

Defibrillation is the first treatment for cardiac arrest, followed by epinephrine if three attempts at defibrillation fail. You should also oxygenate the patient.

If defibrillation isn't available, perform cardiopulmonary resuscitation until advanced cardiac life-support measures become available.

Cardiac muscle dysfunction

MI may cause several types of cardiac muscle dysfunction, depending on the area of damage of the myocardium. (See *Cardiac muscle dysfunction: Signs and symptoms.*)

My poor, ruptured ventricular septum. It may lead to heart failure or cardiogenic shock.

Ventricular septal defect

In a septal wall MI, the ventricular septum can rupture, producing a ventricular septal defect. A septal defect may occur soon after the MI or up to 1 week later. It may cause heart failure and cardiogenic shock and may lead to death.

A ventricular septal defect may be treated with diuretics, inotropic drugs, vasodilators, intra-aortic balloon counterpulsation, or surgery to repair the septal wall.

Ventricular wall rupture

A large ventricular MI can cause a ventricle wall to rupture, leading to cardiac tamponade and death. If the patient survives, surgery is necessary to repair the wall.

Cardiac muscle dysfunction: Signs and symptoms

Ventricular septal defect
- Heart failure
- Cardiogenic shock
- New murmur at the left sternal border between the fourth and fifth intercostal spaces
- Chest pain
- Hypotension
- Atrioventricular block

Ventricular wall rupture
- Sudden tearing pain
- Hypotension
- Distended neck veins
- Pulseless electrical activity

Ventricular aneurysm
- Heart failure
- Ventricular arrhythmias
- Arterial emboli
- Double or displaced apical impulse

Papillary muscle rupture
- Chest pain
- Dyspnea
- Fatigue
- Tachycardia
- Systolic murmur

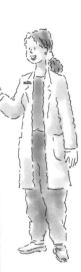

Ventricular aneurysm

An inferior or anterior MI can result in a ventricular aneurysm hours, days, weeks, or even months after the MI. Treatment may include anticoagulants to dissolve the thrombus, measures to control heart failure and arrhythmias, or surgical resection.

Papillary muscle rupture

Papillary muscle rupture can occur during an MI or the first week of recovery. A rupture of this kind often affects the mitral valve, leaving the valve loose and ineffective. This patient may require valve repair or replacement.

Cardiogenic shock

Lack of blood flow during an MI can damage the myocardium of the left ventricle, causing the ventricle to function poorly. This can result in cardiogenic shock, a complication that affects 10% to 20% of patients with acute MI. Without proper treatment, it can lead to death.

Look for hypotension, impaired consciousness...

Signs and symptoms of cardiogenic shock result from the heart's inability to pump blood efficiently throughout the body. Look for:
- cold, clammy skin
- elevated pulmonary artery pressure and pulmonary artery wedge pressure
- hypotension
- impaired consciousness
- low cardiac output
- pulmonary congestion
- peripheral edema
- tachycardia
- urine output less than 20 ml/hour.

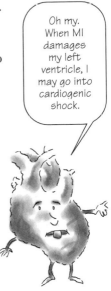

Oh my. When MI damages my left ventricle, I may go into cardiogenic shock.

Treat with fluids, vasopressors...

Treatment usually includes administration of I.V. fluids and vasopressors such as dobutamine to increase blood pressure and improve cardiac output. The patient may also need intubation to maintain his airway and improve oxygenation.

If the condition persists, the patient may need an intra-aortic balloon pump to improve coronary blood flow and reduce afterload.

GI complications

GI complications can result from an MI, from its treatment, or from lack of activity after an MI.

Check for nausea, vomiting, distention...

Analgesics and other medications used to treat MI may cause nausea and vomiting. Preventing vomiting, which may lead to arrhythmias, is especially important.

Abdominal distention, constipation, and fecal impaction can develop after an MI because of:

• decreased activity
• decreased dietary fiber intake
• medication such as morphine, beta blockers, or angiotensin-converting enzyme (ACE) inhibitors
• potassium depletion by diuretics.

Treat with antiemetics, fiber, fluid...

Treat vomiting with an antiemetic. To help relieve other GI problems, provide fiber and fluid and encourage the patient to increase activity when appropriate.

Also, because anxiety may provoke GI dysfunction, teach the patient relaxation techniques.

Heart failure

This dangerous complication occurs when the heart can't pump enough blood to meet the body's metabolic needs. The severity of heart failure depends on the amount of damage the MI causes in the left ventricle. Heart failure accounts for one-third of all MI deaths.

> How severe is the patient's heart failure? That depends on how much damage the MI caused my left ventricle.

Assess for fluid overload, fatigue...

Be alert for the following signs and symptoms of heart failure:
- dyspnea and possibly respiratory failure
- fatigue and weakness
- fluid overload as indicated by edema, elevated pulmonary artery wedge pressure, neck vein distention, or crackles
- low cardiac output
- confusion
- S_3 or S_4 heart sounds.

Treat with ACE inhibitor or digoxin...

Expect to give a drug that improves the heart's pumping action, such as an ACE inhibitor or digoxin. To remove excess fluid, plan to administer a diuretic and re-

strict the patient's sodium and fluid intake.

When the patient is stable and dis-
charged from the hospital, he may receive carvedilol (Coreg), a beta blocker.

Mitral insufficiency

The valve most commonly affected by an
MI is the mitral valve. In mitral insufficiency, the valve fails to close properly
during ventricular systole, causing the
left ventricle to pump blood into the aorta
and backwards into the left atrium.

Overfilled atrium

In a patient with mitral insufficiency, left
atrial pressure increases and pulmonary
edema develops. This can quickly lead to
acute pulmonary edema and death.

Look for dyspnea, orthopnea...

To detect mitral insufficiency, notice the following signs and symptoms:
- dyspnea
- orthopnea
- palpitations
- paroxysmal nocturnal dyspnea

A patient with
mitral
insufficiency
is at risk for
pulmonary
edema.

• weakness.

Treat with mechanical ventilation, valve repair...

Prepare the patient for mechanical ventilation or possible intra-aortic balloon counterpulsation until the valve can be surgically repaired. Administer a vasodilator as prescribed to reduce cardiac afterload and relieve symptoms.

How irritating! Debris from a damaged myocardium may inflame the sac that surrounds me!

Pericarditis

Pericarditis is an inflammation of the sac that surrounds the heart. The initial irritation usually stems from debris and other exudates from the damaged myocardium. Pericarditis may persist for up to 3 months after an MI.

Watch for chest pain, fever...

Watch for the signs and symptoms of pericarditis, including:
• atypical, long-lasting chest pain
• chest pain that increases when the patient breathes deeply or leans forward
• elevated erythrocyte sedimentation rate
• low-grade fever

• pericardial friction rub
• ST-segment elevation in leads facing the inflammation.

Treat with analgesics and anti-inflammatories

Treat with analgesics to reduce chest pain and anti-inflammatory drugs to reduce the swelling of the heart sac.

Thromboembolism

MI may cause a thrombus to form in several places in the body. Thrombus formation in the left ventricle can lead to systemic embolism. Thrombi in deep leg veins usually produce pulmonary embolism.

Look for fever, pain, swelling...

Assess the patient for the following signs and symptoms:
• hemiparesis (when cerebral circulation is involved)
• hypertension (if renal circulation becomes compromised)
• fever
• pain and swelling in an arm or leg
• redness in an arm or leg.

Treat with anticoagulants, movement...

Treat a thromboembolism with anticoagulants. To reduce swelling, apply warm compresses. Encourage the patient to ambulate to prevent thromboembolism from forming in the extremities, and apply antiembolism stockings as needed.

Quick quiz

1. After an MI, the most common complication is:

    A. arrhythmia.

    B. heart failure.

    C. cardiac arrest.

Answer: A. Arrhythmia is the most common post-MI complication. PVC is the most common type of arrhythmia.

2. Treatment of heart failure after an MI usually does *not* include:

    A. ACE inhibitors.

    B. digoxin.

    C. calcium channel blockers.

Answer: C. ACE inhibitors and digoxin are more commonly used than calcium channel blockers to treat heart failure.

3. GI complications of an MI can result from:
- A. fluid overload.
- B. excessive activity post-MI.
- C. adverse drug reactions.

Answer: C. Adverse reactions to drugs, such as analgesics, used to treat MI may cause GI complications— for example, nausea and vomiting. Damage from the MI itself and lack of activity after an MI may also cause GI complications.

Scoring

☆☆☆ If you answered all three questions correctly, stupendous! Clearly the complications of MI aren't too complicated for you.

☆☆ If you answered two questions correctly, right on! You've got the right rhythm for this chapter.

☆ If you answered fewer than two questions correctly, have no fear. Studying the chapter again should prevent further complications.

6

Teaching patients with MI

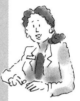

Key facts
- During your teaching session, explain to the patient that chest pain results when the heart doesn't receive enough oxygen.
- Your teaching should cover diagnostic tests and the significance of results to the patient, lifestyle changes that may help prevent another MI, a thorough explanation of medications, and a description of procedures and treatments.
- The patient will be able to resume activity in consultation with his primary care provider but he'll need to build toward more taxing activities.
- Teach the patient to follow a low-fat, low-cholesterol diet.

Teaching about the disorder

Suffering an MI is a frightening experience. Teaching the patient about his disorder, his diagnosis, and ways he can help himself recover will help him become more confident about managing his condition. Plus, it provides support and gives him an opportunity to express his concerns. Educating his family also helps the patient establish a support system.

The basics

Begin by explaining to the patient that the heart depends on the coronary arteries for its blood supply. When the blood supply decreases or ceases, a part of the heart receives no oxygen and the tissue dies. This condition is known as a myocardial infarction, often called an MI or heart attack.

The usual suspect

Tell the patient that the most common cause of this decreased blood supply is atherosclerosis. In atherosclerosis, fatty plaques form along the lining of the coronary arteries, blocking blood flow to the heart.

Pain? A sign of insufficient oxygen

Explain to the patient that chest pain is a common symptom of MI. Chest pain results when the heart doesn't receive enough oxygen.

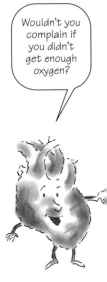

Wouldn't you complain if you didn't get enough oxygen?

In addition, explain that these signs and symptoms may also result from an MI:
- a feeling of impending doom
- left-sided chest pain
- midscapular pain
- pain radiating to the arms, back, or shoulders
- palpitations, cold sweat, paleness
- shortness of breath or difficulty breathing.

Teaching about tests

Teach the patient that diagnostic tests are performed to confirm MI and assess damage to his heart.

Confirming MI

Teach the patient that:
- An ECG is a noninvasive test that reveals heart rhythm changes or areas with a decreased oxygen supply.
- A blood test is used to measure cardiac enzymes, which helps determine if his heart has suffered damage.

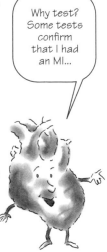

Why test? Some tests confirm that I had an MI...

Assessing damage

Other tests reveal the extent of damage to the heart, such as:

• cardiac catheterization, a test in which a small catheter is inserted into the groin area and threaded up the aorta to the coronary arteries

• echocardiogram, a noninvasive test that reveals heart wall movement

• exercise ECG, which evaluates the heart's response to walking on a tread-mill and identifies if ischemia has occurred

• radionuclide imaging, a test in which an injected substance shows heart damage on film.

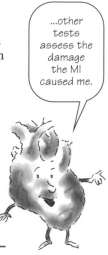

...other tests assess the damage the MI caused me.

Teaching about medication

To encourage the patient to comply with his medication regimen, explain each drug thoroughly. Answer all of the patient's (and caregivers') questions, and instruct him to call his primary care provider before taking any over-the-counter medications.

No place like home

Stay on schedule

To help the patient comply with his medication regimen at home, help him establish a daily medication routine that fits his lifestyle.

Because high blood pressure increases his risk of having another MI, also teach the patient how to take his pulse and use a self-monitoring blood pressure device.

How much, how often, how it interacts

For each medication, be sure to tell the patient the:

- amount of medication to take
- timing of doses
- adverse reactions
- interactions with other drugs.

Remind the patient never to stop taking a medication abruptly without notifying his primary care provider. Also tell him to report any adverse reactions and teach him about the specific kind of medication he'll be taking. (See *Stay on schedule.*)

Thrombolytics

Inform the patient that thrombolytics dissolve the thrombus occluding the coronary artery and allow blood flow to return to the heart.

Tell me if it hurts

Teach the patient:
• that he will be closely monitored throughout the infusion
• to report any adverse reactions, especially chest pain.

Beta-adrenergic blockers

If the patient is taking a beta-adrenergic blocker, tell him:
• that this medication helps lower heart rate and blood pressure, which reduces the heart's workload
• to protect the medication from direct sunlight
• to swallow the beta-adrenergic blocker directly — never break, crush, or chew it
• to call his primary care provider if he experiences adverse reactions (never just stop taking the drug)
• to monitor his pulse and blood pressure
• to withhold the drug and call his primary care provider if his heart

> Make sure the patient understands why he's taking a beta-adrenergic blocker: to reduce the heart's workload.

rate falls below the rate specified by the primary care provider.

Aspirin

Teach the patient that aspirin works as a blood thinner, which improves blood flow in the coronary arteries. Tell him to:

• take his aspirin at the same time each day

• avoid taking aspirin at any other time because it may make his blood too thin

• report any unusual bleeding or bruising to his primary care provider.

ACE inhibitors

Explain to the patient that angiotensin-converting enzyme (ACE) inhibitors block the conversion of the enzyme angiotensin I to angiotensin II. This relaxes the arteries and reduces strain on the heart.

Rate, pressure, studies

Because of these effects, remind the patient to monitor his heart rate and blood pressure regularly. Because these medications may also affect his potassium, creati-

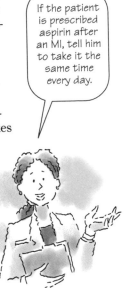

If the patient is prescribed aspirin after an MI, tell him to take it the same time every day.

nine, and blood urea nitrogen levels, he should come in for laboratory studies as directed by his primary care provider.

Also discuss with the patient whether his ACE inhibitor needs to be taken on an empty stomach.

Nitroglycerin

Teach the patient that nitroglycerin decreases the heart's workload by reducing the amount of blood the heart has to pump and reducing blood pressure.

Nitroglycerin is often prescribed to treat chest pain. (See *When pain strikes.*)

Handle with care

Explain to the patient that nitroglycerin needs to be handled carefully to ensure its effectiveness. Tell him that nitroglycerin:

• reacts to light and should always be kept in a dark place

• reacts to plastic and metal and should, therefore, always be kept in a glass bottle

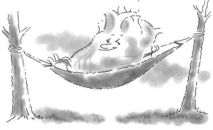

Nitroglycerin eases my workload by reducing the amount of blood I have to pump. Thanks for the rest.

Listen up!

When pain strikes

Nitroglycerin is often used to treat chest pain. Tell the patient to follow these guidelines if chest pain occurs:
• Try to relieve the pain by resting.
• If pain is unrelieved, continue to rest and take one nitroglycerin
tablet every 5 minutes (he should take no more than three tablets
total).
• If the chest pain isn't relieved by sublingual nitroglycerin, call 911
and wait for assistance; tell the patient not to drive to the hospital.

Stick it here

Most patients take nitroglycerin sublingually but some use a nitroglycerin patch.
   If your patient will use the patch, tell him to:
• remove the backing
• apply the patch to a nonhairy part of the body
• remove the old patch before applying a new one
• remember to change sites for the patch.

• reacts to moisture so it should never
be kept in the bathroom
• degrades with heat and shouldn't be
carried directly against the body but
should be placed in an empty pill bottle
before carrying it in a shirt pocket
• should always fizz when placed under
the tongue and, if not, may have degrad-
ed and lost its effectiveness.

Also make sure that the patient knows to check the expiration date. Remind him that his prescription should be refilled every 6 months.

Antiarrhythmics

Teach the patient that antiarrhythmics work to restore the heart rhythm to a normal pattern.

Even at night

Instruct the patient to:
• take the drug exactly as prescribed, even if this requires a nighttime dose
• monitor blood pressure and heart rate
• return for routine blood tests to monitor medication and electrolyte levels.

Adrenergics

Explain to the patient that adrenergics increase the heart's pumping ability.

We'll keep an eye on you

Teach the patient that he:
• must have a health care professional closely monitor his heart rate and rhythm, blood pressure, and urine output while he's receiving this medication

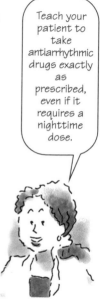

Teach your patient to take antiarrhythmic drugs exactly as prescribed, even if it requires a nighttime dose.

• may need to receive this medication through a central I.V. line, which the doctor will insert

• should report any adverse reactions, such as dizziness and palpitations.

Morphine

Inform the patient that morphine should relieve his chest pain. It also decreases the heart's need for oxygen.

Tell him that his blood pressure will be closely monitored while he's taking this drug. Also tell him to immediately report any chest pain.

Thanks to morphine, I'll get by with less oxygen.

Diuretics

Explain to the patient that diuretics reduce fluid in the body. This can lower blood pressure and reduce the heart's workload.

Fatigue at first

Tell the patient that he may feel tired when he first begins this medication. Also tell him that:

• the medication can cause dizziness or light-headedness

• he should report adverse reactions such as leg cramps, irregular heart rate, or confusion.

By compressing plaque against the vessel wall, PTCA opens the patient's blocked artery.

Teaching about procedures

Explain to the patient that percutaneous transluminal coronary angioplasty (PTCA) is the most common procedure used to treat MI.

Teach him that PTCA improves coronary artery blood flow by opening a blocked or narrowed artery. Explain that a balloon-tipped catheter compresses cholesterol deposits against the arterial wall, widening the diameter of the artery.

Lean back and relax

After the procedure, tell the patient to immediately report chest pain and expect:

• frequent monitoring of vital signs, fluid status, the insertion site, and peripheral pulses

• to drink fluids

• to maintain bed rest, with the head of the bed no higher than 15 degrees. (See *Post-PTCA points.*)

No place like home

Post-PTCA points

To prepare the patient to go home after percutaneous transluminal coronary angioplasty (PTCA), include these points in your discharge teaching.

• Limit activity as ordered.
• Don't lift more than 10 lb (4.5 kg) for 2 to 3 weeks.
• Apply pressure over the insertion site when coughing or sneezing.
• Don't bear down when having a bowel movement.
• If bleeding occurs, apply pressure to the site for 15 to 20 minutes.
• If bleeding is severe, notify the primary care provider or go to the hospital.

You're not out of the woods yet

Explain to the patient that reocclusion may occur, despite the procedure. Tell him that if reocclusion doesn't occur during the first 6 months, the prognosis is usually good if the patient continues his drug regimen and adopts a healthy lifestyle, including proper diet and exercise.

Teaching about surgery

Tell the patient that coronary artery by-pass graft (CABG) surgery is the most common surgery to treat MI. Explain that a CABG bypasses the blockage in a coronary artery, restoring blood flow to the heart. During surgery, the doctor removes part of a healthy vessel (usually the saphenous vein or mammary artery) and grafts it above and below the blocked coronary artery. Circulation then passes through the graft.

Got a blockage? Bypass it. CABG allows blood to get past a blocked artery.

Chest tube, catheter, cough pillow

After surgery, explain the monitoring devices to the patient and tell him that his vital signs, dressings, and tubes will be checked frequently. Inform him that he:

• will have his chest tubes removed 1 to 3 days after surgery

• may have a catheter in his neck to monitor his heart pressures, which should be removed 1 to 2 days after surgery

• will be connected to a machine to help him breathe but will be removed as soon as he can breathe on his own
• will be assisted out of bed the day after his surgery
• should plan to go home 4 to 7 days after surgery (see *Surgery send-off*)
• may feel somewhat depressed for up to several weeks after surgery
• should wear antiembolism stockings to promote circulation in his legs
• should use his incentive spirometer as prescribed

• should use his cough pillow to support his chest when he coughs

• should request pain medication when needed.

Teaching about lifestyle changes

You can help the patient prevent future MIs by teaching him about lifestyle changes, including:
• resuming activities and exercise
• eating a heart-healthy diet
• quitting smoking
• reducing stress.

Activity and exercise

Inform the patient that he'll be able to resume activity in consultation with his primary care provider but that he'll need to build toward more taxing activities.

Thanks to exercise, I can work more efficiently.

A bundle of benefits

Explain to the patient that while exercise doesn't guarantee that he won't suffer another MI, it offers many potential benefits. Exercise can:
• condition the heart to work more efficiently
• increase high-density lipoprotein levels
• lower triglyceride levels
• improve blood glucose levels
• control weight
• reduce anxiety and depression.

Making whoopee

Also discuss any concerns the patient might have about resuming sexual activity. (See *Let's talk about sex,* page 132.)

Diet

Teach the patient to follow a low-fat, low-cholesterol diet. Provide him with low-fat recipes, and urge him to stay away from prepackaged foods, such as convenience foods, that are high in fat and cholesterol.

Teach the patient how to read food labels to avoid foods that are high in fat and sodium. Also encourage him to plan ahead for special meals,

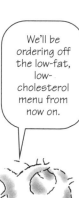

We'll be ordering off the low-fat, low-cholesterol menu from now on.

Listen up!

Let's talk about sex

Many patients feel concerned about resuming sexual activity after an MI. Discuss resuming sexual activity with the patient, explaining that he should:
• take a relatively passive role in sex to avoid overstressing his heart
• plan sexual activity for when he's well rested, such as in the morning
• wait for 2 hours after a meal before engaging in intercourse
• take nitroglycerin before intercourse.

such as birthdays, anniversaries, and holidays, and adjust his other meals if he expects the menu for these events to include high-fat items. (See *What's on the menu?*)

Smoking

Explain to a patient who smokes that nicotine narrows the coronary arteries. It also roughens the linings of those arteries, making it easier for plaque to build.

What's on the menu?

A typical menu, per day, for a post-MI patient might include:
- 2 to 4 servings of fruits
- 3 to 5 servings of vegetables
- 2 servings of lean protein
- 4 to 6 servings of breads, cereals, pasta, and starchy vegetables
- 2 to 4 servings of fat-free milk and low-fat dairy products
- 1 to 2 servings of fat.

What's a serving?

Explain to the patient that he might define a serving for each group as:
- fruit and vegetables: 1 medium-sized piece of fruit, ¾ cup of fruit or vegetable juice, 1 cup raw leafy vegetable, or ½ cup cooked vegetables
- protein: ½ chicken breast (skin removed), 2 thin slices of roast beef, or ¾ can of tuna fish
- breads, cereals, pasta: 1 slice of bread, ½ bagel or muffin, 1 cup of flaked cereal, ½ cup of pasta or other cooked grains, or ½ cup of potatoes
- dairy: 1 cup skim milk, 1 cup nonfat yogurt, 1 oz low-fat cheese, or ½ cup low-fat cottage cheese
- fats: 1 tsp vegetable oil or margarine, 1 tbs salad dressing, 2 tsp mayonnaise or peanut butter.

Individual approach

Methods used to quit smoking depend on the individual patient and the level of his addiction. If the patient has a low dependence on nicotine, then group therapy, hypnosis, or acupuncture can prove beneficial.

Gum or patch?

For patients with a higher degree of addiction, nicotine replacement therapy (in the form of gum or patches) may be used, either alone or together with other methods.

Bupropion (Wellbutrin) is an antidepressant that may decrease the patient's craving for nicotine when used alone or with group therapy.

Stress

Tell the patient that stress tends to increase the likelihood of heart disease. Teach him about ways to reduce stress such as:

• taking 15 to 20 minutes per day to sit quietly and breathe deeply
• exercising regularly
• limiting caffeine and alcohol intake
• meditating and using other relaxation techniques.

Chill out. Stress tends to increase the likelihood of heart disease.

A few final words

Explain that although the MI has caused permanent damage to the patient's heart, he can improve his overall health and reduce his risk of having another MI. To do this, he needs to modify his risk factors and follow his treatment regimen.

Stay on track

Remind him to take his medications as prescribed, and keep his nitroglycerin with him at all times. Also urge him to get a flu shot yearly.

Encourage him to follow his primary care provider's orders for an exercise program and for other lifestyle changes. Also encourage the patient to call the primary care provider with any questions. He can also learn more about his condition at the library or from sources on the Internet.

Pick up the phone

Finally, make the patient aware of the signs of a recurrent MI. Tell him to notify his primary care provider if he feels:

- anxiety
- chest pain

Learning about MI on the Internet

The following directory lists some key Web sites that offer information about myocardial infarction (MI) and its treatment.

American Heart Association

http://www.amhrt.org/warning.html

This site provides a brief overview of MI for patients. It discusses warning signs and symptoms of an MI, tells what an MI is, describes what to do in an emergency, and offers a health risk awareness quiz.

Heart Point

http://www.heartpoint.com/mimore.html

Presented in a question-and-answer format, this site provides an excellent overview for patients. It discusses the causes, symptoms, risk factors, and effects of an MI. It also presents information about medications, cholesterol levels, bypass surgery, balloon procedures, ways to prevent another MI, and more.

Mayo Health Clinic

http://www.mayohealth.org

From the home page, you can link to Mayo Clinic health sites that address questions about MI. Links enable the user to access information about causes of MI, prevention of MI, the relationship of MI to cholesterol levels and diet, medications for MI, and more. The site also gives definitions of complex words. It's good for patients and health care providers.

National Library of Medicine

http://medlineplus.nlm.nih.gov/medlineplus/heartattack.html

The National Library of Medicine's MEDLINEplus information pages direct patients to resources that provide answers to health questions.

- diaphoresis
- nausea
- radiating pain to the back, neck, left arm, or jaw.

Quick quiz

1. If your patient must take nitroglycerin, you should instruct him:

    A. to take one every 5 minutes if he feels chest pain.

    B. to keep it in the bathroom cabinet.

    C. to keep it in a clear plastic box.

Answer: A. Teach the patient to take nitroglycerin every 5 minutes for chest pain (up to a maximum of three).

2. After an MI, beta-adrenergic blockers are valuable because they:

    A. decrease the strength of the heart's contraction.

    B. decrease heart rate and blood pressure.

    C. can prevent heart failure.

Answer: B. Beta-adrenergic blockers reduce stress on the myocardium by slowing the heart rate and lowering blood pressure.

3. For a patient who has just had CABG surgery, you should teach him to expect all of the following, except:

A. hospitalization for 2 more weeks.

B. assistance out of bed the first day.

C. a chest tube.

Answer: A. After CABG, patients usually go home in 4 to 7 days.

Scoring

☆☆☆ If you answered three questions correctly, incredible! You've indicated indispensable insight into MI instruction.

☆☆ If you answered fewer than three questions correctly, don't worry. Every good teacher knows that review is important.

Index

i refers to an illustration; t refers to a table.

i refers to an illustration; t refers to a table.

i refers to an illustration; t refers to a table.

i refers to an illustration; t refers to a table.

i refers to an illustration; t refers to a table.

i refers to an illustration; t refers to a table.